Psychiatric Services in Jails and Prisons

A Task Force Report of the American Psychiatric Association

Second Edition

The American Psychiatric Association Task Force to Revise the APA Guidelines on Psychiatric Services in Jails and Prisons

Henry C. Weinstein, M.D., *Chair*

Kathryn A. Burns, M.D., M.P.H.

Cassandra F. Newkirk, M.D.

John S. Zil, M.D., M.P.H., J.D.

Joel A. Dvoskin, Ph.D., *Consultant*

Henry J. Steadman, Ph.D., *Consultant*

Psychiatric Services in Jails and Prisons

A Task Force Report of the American Psychiatric Association

Second Edition

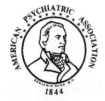

Published by the American Psychiatric Association
Washington, D.C.

Note: The authors have worked to ensure that all information in this book concerning drug dosages, schedules, and routes of administration is accurate as of the time of publication and consistent with standards set by the U.S. Food and Drug Administration and the general medical community. As medical research and practice advance, however, therapeutic standards may change. For this reason and because human and mechanical errors sometimes occur, we recommend that readers follow the advice of a physician who is directly involved in their care or the care of a member of their family.

The findings, opinions, and conclusions of this report do not necessarily represent the views of the officers, trustees, all members of the task force, or all members of the American Psychiatric Association. Task force reports are considered a substantive contribution of the ongoing analysis and evaluation of problems, programs, issues, and practices in a given area of concern.

Copyright © 2000 American Psychiatric Association
ALL RIGHTS RESERVED
Manufactured in the United States of America on acid-free paper
03 02 01   4 3 2
First Edition

American Psychiatric Association
1400 K Street, N.W., Washington, DC 20005
www.psych.org

Library of Congress Cataloging-in-Publication Data
American Psychiatric Association. Task Force to Revise the APA Guidelines on Psychiatric Services in Jails and Prisons.
   Psychiatric services in jails and prisons: a task force report of the American Psychiatric Association / American Psychiatric Association, Task Force to Revise the APA Guidelines on Psychiatric Services in Jails and Prisons ; Henry C. Weinstein, chair . . . [et al.].—2nd ed.
      p.   ; cm.
   Earlier edition prepared by American Psychiatric Association. Task Force on Psychiatric Services in Jails and Prisons.
   Includes bibliographical references and index.
   ISBN 0-89042-287-7 (alk. paper)
   1. Prisoners—Mental health services—Standards. I. Weinstein, Henry C. II. Title.
   [DNLM: 1. Mental Health Services—organization & administration—United States. 2. Delivery of Health Care—organization & administration—United States. Prisons—United States. 4. Psychotherapy—organization & administration—United States. WM 30 A52285p 2000]
RC451.4.P68 A44 2000
365'.66—dc21

                                                          99-050098

British Library Cataloguing in Publication Data
A CIP record is available from the British Library.

Contents

Contributors

Kathryn A. Burns, M.D., M.P.H.
Director, Forensic Services, Twin Valley Psychiatric System—Columbus Campus, Columbus, Ohio; Assistant Clinical Professor of Psychiatry, Case Western Reserve University School of Medicine, Cleveland, Ohio; Wright State University School of Medicine, Dayton, Ohio; University of Cincinnati College of Medicine, Cincinnati, Ohio; Ohio State University School of Medicine, Columbus, Ohio

Joel A. Dvoskin, Ph.D., A.B.P.P. (Forensic)
University of Arizona College of Law; University of Arizona College of Medicine; New York University School of Medicine, New York, New York

Cassandra F. Newkirk, M.D.
Chair, American Psychiatric Association Consortium on Special Delivery Settings (representing jails and prisons) of the Council on Psychiatric Services; Monitor of mental health services in several prison litigation cases; Consultant for National Institution of Corrections technical assistance grants in women's prisons

Henry J. Steadman, Ph.D.
President, Policy Research Associates, Delmar, New York

Henry C. Weinstein, M.D.
Director, Program in Psychiatry and the Law, New York University Medical Center; Clinical Professor of Psychiatry, New York University School of Medicine, New York, New York

John S. Zil, M.D., M.P.H., J.D.
Chief Psychiatrist, California Department of Corrections; Legislative Liaison, University of California

Foreword

The idea of public service is so deeply ingrained in the practice of medicine that we rarely think about it or acknowledge it. We certainly don't discuss it as such.

Medicine is a paradigmatic "calling." Many physicians have known that they would become "doctors" from an early age. And, I've found, many have started to "practice" early—listening to, trying to understand, and trying to help their friends and others. At best, this leads to the development of what we later notice is this young person's "bedside manner": how he or she relates and communicates with another person—the patient. This ineffable contact, we have known for thousands of years, may be a critical factor in the "treatment."

The satisfaction derived from this "work" is, at times, hard to describe. It imbues in the physician, I believe, a special, complex sense of responsibility and often drives him or her to seek to help the most unfortunate, the neediest, and certainly the least able to afford a fee.

But what is it that drives a physician to treat an inmate in a prison? Is it that, in addition to the satisfaction and responsibility described above, these men and women, having been cast out, are truly society's "outcasts"? And then, to seek out and treat the criminally insane? Is it the challenge or is it the gratification of actually helping—of bringing the best to those many regard as the worst?

This need and drive to help in public service has a long tradition in psychiatry. Benjamin Rush, regarded as the first American psychiatrist and the founder of the American Psychiatric Association, wrote extensively on the treatment of deviant behavior. American psychiatry's concern has always been with the criminal and with the study of the criminal as an individual.

The American Psychiatric Association has continued this tradition. Selected recent activities of the American Psychiatric Association in providing care to those in jails and prisons are summarized in the appendix to this report. These guidelines stand for this deep commitment, in the public service, to treat the mentally ill in jails and prisons: to actively seek them out and give them the best—the best that we can.

It has been just 10 years since the first edition of these guidelines was approved by the Board of Directors of the American Psychiatric Association. Now, at the dawn of a new millennium, the American Psychiatric Association presents the revised, second edition of these guidelines and salutes our members who carry on this special, particularly noble, tradition of public service.

Henry C. Weinstein, M.D.
November 15, 1999

Preface

For the past decade, the first edition of these unique guidelines, known as the American Psychiatric Association (APA) Guidelines for Psychiatric Services in Jails and Prisons, has lighted the way for those seeking to navigate the perilous shoals of providing psychiatric services in jails and prisons. These guidelines have been used and cited extensively in many contexts. They have been used in educational contexts for the teaching and training of correctional mental health professionals, cited as a reference for certifying examinations, used for planning and improving mental health services in jails and prisons, and frequently quoted in litigation. They also have been used by surveyors and monitors of correctional facilities.

Since the publication of the first edition in 1989, American jails and prisons have seen many changes, including considerable litigation, the development of consumer groups, dramatic increases in census, and the creation of some exemplary programs. In the administration of mental health services in jails and prisons, there has been a marked shift toward privatization, and some jurisdictions are experimenting with fee-for-service or copayment plans.

It has been a decade of marked interest and dramatic change. The National Commission on Correctional Health Care, with the active participation of the representatives of the APA, continued its leadership role, with new provisions in its groundbreaking and forward-looking standards for the care and treatment of the mentally ill.

Other accrediting organizations, such as the American Correctional Association and the Joint Commission on the Accreditation of Healthcare Organizations, have also begun to focus some welcome attention on correctional mental health care.

Most important for psychiatry, the Accreditation Council on Graduate Medical Education, with the active participation of members of the APA, in response to the recognition of the subspecialty of forensic psychiatry, has developed criteria for fellowship training programs in forensic psychiatry that require a substantial correctional psychiatry component. This development ensures the interest of academic psychiatry in correctional psychiatry and the encouraging and nurturing of future correctional psychiatrists.

The preface to the first edition of these guidelines, the 1989 Report of the Task Force on Psychiatric Services in Jails and Prisons, stated that "[t]he Task Force sees the publication of these principles and guidelines as 'work in progress' and expects them to be revised in accordance with experience in their utilization and further refinement in evaluation and review techniques" (p. 1). This second edition seeks to carry out that expectation, and the time clearly is propitious for a new edition of this work and a reconsideration of these principles and guidelines.

Again, the Task Force wishes to express its gratitude to all those whose help has been so important in this work. We especially are grateful to the Council on Psychiatric Services and its chairpersons, who have been so supportive during the course of the Task Force's work. Certain people deserve special mention. Dr. Richard Fields, when he was Chair of the Council on Psychiatric Services, provided the understanding, encouragement, energy, and enthusiasm that led to the creation of this Task Force. We wish also to acknowledge Dr. Roger Peele, present Chair of the Council, whose support in the governance of the APA for the interests of correctional psychiatrists continues to inspire and motivate our efforts.

We would also like to take this opportunity to thank all the APA staff who have been so critical to these efforts. Corky Hart has been a rock of support for this Task Force as well as the original Task Force and its successor, the APA Committee on Psychiatric Services in Jails and Prisons. Katherine Chambless and Lisa Fields, more recent members of our staff support network, have given unstintingly of their best efforts.

Our reviewers have been especially generous with their time, and their comments have stimulated our discussions and our efforts. A number of them have made considerable efforts on our behalf. Dr. Jaye Anno's detailed and thoughtful review was an inspiration. Dr. Thomas Grisso's careful analysis of this work assisted in many of our most difficult deliberations.

We also wish to thank our colleagues Drs. Carl Bell, Bill Buzogany, Dennis Koson, Jeffrey Metzner, Ray Patterson, and Bob Phillips.

We thank our other reviewers, Cheryl Al-Mateen, M.D., Ray Coleman, Wendy Edwards, Steve Ingley, Ledro Justice, M.D., Hal Smith, and Lois Ventura, Ph.D.

The Task Force acknowledges with gratitude that it received partial support for this revision from the National GAINS Center for People With Co-Occurring Disorders in the Justice System.

The members of the Task Force wish to take this opportunity to acknowledge with gratitude and affection the enormous efforts of our consultants, Drs. Joel A. Dvoskin and Henry J. Steadman.

Finally, the Task Force wishes to dedicate this edition of these guidelines to the memory of Saleem Shah. Dr. Shah, a psychologist and member of the Task Force that created the first edition of these guidelines, was a friend and a man who personified the essence of interdisciplinary collegiality and cooperation that is so necessary to bring about the best possible professional care and concern for patients in correctional facilities.

We are all *potentially* such sick men. The sanest and best of us are of one clay with the lunatics and prison-mates.

William James
The Varieties of Religious Experience (1902)

Introduction

In September of 1989, when the first edition of these guidelines was published, an editorial in *The American Journal of Psychiatry* noted, "On any day, our nation's jails and prisons hold an estimated 1.2 million men and women." Ten years later, this number is now 1.8 million.

Over the last 15 years, the U.S. jail population has increased from 221,815 to 567,079—an increase of 156%. More importantly, in 1993, the most recent year for which data are available, nearly 10 million people were booked into these 3,304 jails. During the same time period, the federal and state prison population exploded from 744,208 in 1985 to 1,725,842 in 1997—an increase of 132%.

Clearly, the major causes of these huge increases were harsher sanctions associated with the "war on drugs" and the general public's attitude toward "getting tough on crime." In addition, more rigid sentencing policies removed discretion from judges on sentence lengths and limited parole board discretion in the release of inmates.

Many studies have consistently demonstrated that about 20% of inmates in jails and prisons have serious mental illnesses and are in need of psychiatric care. Up to 5% are actively psychotic.

The question is, with upward of 700,000 men and women entering the U.S. criminal justice system each year with active symptoms of serious mental disorders, with 75% of these people having co-occurring substance abuse disorders, and with these persons likely to stay incarcerated four to five times longer than similarly charged persons without mental disorders, what are our duties and responsibilities? This is the question to which this document is addressed. How do we live up to our personal moral principles, our professional ethics, and our public service obligations in the face of these overwhelming numbers?

This document is intended both to prod to action and to provide comprehensive guidance on how to fulfill these responsibilities to ourselves, our profession, and these badly underserved patients. We have the technologies for treatment. We have the knowledge and the skills. Yet limited resources and public and professional resistance often impede appropriate response. We believe that this document can help overcome many of these sources of resistance through informed action. It is a belief based on observed quality, humane services, and dedicated practitioners across the United States, that more active involvement of our profession is needed, is possible, and will make a difference.

PART 1

Principles Governing the Delivery of Psychiatric Services in Jails and Prisons

I. Introduction to the Principles

A. Scope

The second edition of the American Psychiatric Association (APA) Guidelines on Psychiatric Services in Jails and Prisons is made up of three major sections. This first section, "Principles Governing the Delivery of Psychiatric Services in Jails and Prisons," presents and discusses the general principles that apply to all types of correctional facilities.[1] The first edition of these guidelines discussed the following principles: quality of care, education and training, consent, confidentiality, treatment, research, administration and administrative issues, and interprofessional relationships. This second edition, in addition to discussing those principles, also covers principles relating to access to care, cultural competence, suicide prevention, ethical issues, and diversion.

The second section, the guidelines themselves ("Guidelines for Psychiatric Services in Jails and Prisons"), sets out, in some detail, the actual services that should be provided in particular settings.

---

[1]For the purposes of these guidelines, *correctional facilities* is a term that includes facilities known as "lockups," which may be under the jurisdiction of the police, as well as jails and prisons. In addition, it should be noted that these guidelines define the term *psychiatric services in jails and prisons* as all mental health services, including substance abuse services, with emphasis on the unique role of psychiatrists in the delivery of these services.

The third section, "Special Applications of the Principles and Guidelines," seeks to apply the principles and guidelines set forth in the first two sections to particular patient populations and to further elaborate on services that should be provided to meet the needs of those particular groups of inmates.

B. The Legal Context

Basic to the understanding of these principles and guidelines is an awareness of the legal context of psychiatric services in jails and prisons. The legal context of providing psychiatric services in jails and prisons is unique. In no other setting are such services constitutionally guaranteed.

Briefly, under the Eighth Amendment of the U.S. Constitution, which prohibits "cruel and unusual punishment," whenever a state or federal governmental entity takes custody of a person, it has a duty to provide for the necessities of life, which the person otherwise is unable to obtain. These include food, clothing, shelter, and medical care. For pretrial detainees, these rights are based on the U.S. Constitution's Fourteenth Amendment guarantee of due process.

A series of decisions since 1976 has established the dimensions and some details of this constitutional guarantee. The U.S. Supreme Court, in the 1976 landmark case *Estelle v. Gamble,* held it unconstitutional for prison officials to be deliberately indifferent to the serious medical needs of those in their custody. *Bowring v. Godwin* (1977) was the first important federal decision to extend this requirement to psychiatric care. Since then, numerous federal and state court decisions have equated medical and psychiatric care, although the Supreme Court has yet to specifically concur.

There have been some very important federal decisions that establish the framework and some specific criteria for constitutionally adequate psychiatric care in jails and prisons. The *Ruiz* decision, a class action suit in Texas (*Ruiz v. Estelle* 1980), listed six explicit criteria for constitutionally acceptable mental health services:

- Systematic screening and evaluation
- Treatment that is more than mere seclusion or close supervision
- Participation by trained mental health professionals
- Accurate, complete, and confidential records

- Safeguards against psychotropic medications that are prescribed in dangerous amounts, without adequate supervision, or otherwise inappropriately administered
- A suicide prevention program

In 1989, *Langley v. Coughlin* listed a number of specific criteria that, if not met, could provide a basis for successful inmate legal claims. Many of these criteria explicitly required providing for so-called secondary or supportive rights, such as taking psychiatric histories and maintaining medical records, in recognition of the fact that such rights are required in order to facilitate the primary right to diagnosis and actual care. *Langley* also explicitly requires that care not be limited to psychotropic medication.

Madrid v. Gomez, in 1995, added several factors that may determine the constitutionality of a correctional mental health system:

- An inmate must have a means of making his or her needs known to the medical staff.
- Sufficient staffing must allow individualized treatment of each inmate with serious mental illness.
- An inmate must have speedy access to services.
- There must be a system of quality assurance.
- Staff must be competent and well trained.
- There must be a system of responding to emergencies and of preventing suicides.

In addition to constitutional mandates, jail and prison mental health services may be required to meet other legal requirements. These include federal laws, such as the Americans With Disabilities Act, and federal regulations, as well as state requirements, established on the basis of state law through constitutions, statutes, and regulations. Services may also be subject to simple tort liability, such as for malpractice.

Finally, an important case for clinicians is the U.S. Supreme Court case of *Youngberg v. Romeo* (1982). Though not a correctional case, *Youngberg* held that professional judgments arrived at and carried out in a professional manner are presumptively constitutional, a principle that has relevance to care in any institutional setting.

II. Access to Mental Health Care and Treatment

A. Adequate and Appropriate Access to Care

"Timely and effective access to mental health treatment is the hallmark of adequate mental health care." This was the fundamental principle of adequate mental health care in jails and prisons set out in the first edition of these guidelines.

To determine whether there is adequate and appropriate access to mental health treatment, the mental health service delivery system must be analyzed to ensure that there are no unreasonable barriers to patients' receiving mental health services. Some examples of unreasonable barriers include instituting or allowing disincentives that would deter a patient from seeking care for his or her legitimate mental health needs; interfering with the prompt transmittal of a patient's oral or written request for care; permitting unreasonable delays before patients are seen by mental health staff or outside consultants; charging fees or imposing costs that prevent or deter patients from seeking care; and, obviously, punishing an inmate for seeking or refusing care.

B. Access to Care in Segregation Units

The difficulties of providing appropriate and adequate access to mental health care and treatment are especially acute in any segregation environment. For the purposes of this document, *segregation* is defined as any unit that confines inmates to their cells 23 or more hours per day. The reasons for such confinement include disciplinary placement and isolation from other inmates for administrative or protective reasons, among others.

In jails and prisons without adequate mental health services, inmates with mental illness often find their way into segregation housing quite unnecessarily, when their mental illness prevents them from understanding or adhering to correctional rules. The recent development of so-called super-max facilities, where inmates may spend years in segregation, thus raises ominous clinical and fairness issues for persons with mental illness.

Thus, one critical barrier to access to mental health care and treatment may occur when an inmate is housed in a segregation environment.

When an inmate is segregated—for any reason—from the general population, the responsibility to address serious mental health needs remains in effect. Indeed, because of the stressful nature of segregation housing, facilities should make special efforts to assess and address mental health treating needs in these settings.

In providing essential mental health service in segregation housing, the following principles should be observed:

- No inmate should be placed in segregation housing solely because he or she exhibits the symptoms of mental illness, unless there is an immediate and serious danger for which there is no other reasonable alternative. (This principle does not refer to medical or psychiatric seclusion, which should follow state mental health law and professional practice.)
- When an inmate is placed in segregated housing for appropriate correctional reasons, the facility remains responsible for meeting all of the serious medical and psychiatric needs of that inmate. Thus, such inmates must receive any mental health services that are deemed essential, their segregation status notwithstanding.
- Inmates who are in current, severe psychiatric crisis, including but not limited to acute psychosis and suicidal depression, should be removed from segregation until such time as they are psychologically able to tolerate that setting.
- Inmates who are known to have serious mental health needs, especially those with a known history of serious and persistent mental illness, when housed in segregation, must be assessed on a regular basis by qualified mental health practitioners, to identify and respond to emerging crises at the earliest possible moment.

Institutions should provide for regular rounds by a qualified mental health clinician in all segregation housing areas. During these rounds, each inmate should be visited briefly so that any emerging problem can be assessed. The clinician should also communicate with segregation security staff in order to identify any inmate who appears to be showing signs of mental deterioration or psychological problems.

The challenge of providing adequate mental health services to inmates in segregation housing is a critical reflection of and a crucial component of a facility's quality of care.

III. Quality of Care

The fundamental policy goal for correctional mental health care is to provide the same level of mental health services to each patient in the criminal justice process that should be available in the community. This policy goal is deliberately higher than the "community standard" that is called for in various legal contexts.

It is imperative that the facility administration be able to gather and assess information relevant to the prevalence of mental illness in the correctional setting, for purposes of needs assessment.

The allocation of resources within a facility is determined by many factors, including the extent of resources available, the size of the facility, the overall organization of the services provided, the mission of the facility, and the lengths of stay of the inmates confined there.

Clearly, the highest priority for care in any institution should be inmates with disruptive symptoms who are severely dangerous. However, similar attention must be paid to those inmates whose suffering, though equally severe, is less obvious or disruptive.

Each facility or administrative authority should have prepared a quality assurance plan that sets out systematically to review and improve the quality of mental health services and the efficiency and effectiveness of the utilization of staff and resources in the delivery of services. Quality assurance activities include credentialing, review of service access and utilization, record keeping and review of records, resource management, morbidity and mortality review, and identification and prevention of risk and the monitoring and review of high-risk critical procedures such as overriding treatment refusals and responding in emergency situations.

Over the past decade a number of organizations have instituted accreditation programs. The accreditation program sponsored by the National Commission on Correctional Health Care is an excellent example. While it generally is appreciated that such accreditation does not guarantee either adequate provision of mental health services or compliance with these guidelines, facilities are encouraged to participate in such programs to further the efforts to enhance the quality of care. Facility administrators and clinicians are also encouraged to become familiar with the standards and guidelines that the Joint Commission on Accreditation of Healthcare Organizations has used to accredit correctional health facilities.

Staffing levels are a particularly thorny and complex subject, because systems vary widely in their organization, physical plants, resource availability, and population characteristics. Nevertheless, concrete statements of such levels are often quite specifically sought by reviewing bodies, such as courts deciding cases and governmental agencies attempting to assess specific budgetary needs and requirements of particular facilities.

Staffing ratios are often sought by courts and regulatory agencies that wish to assert and impose minimally acceptable numbers of staff for each mental health profession. The authors of the first edition of these guidelines were reluctant to specify staffing ratios. They noted that

> we have not sought to specify in detail such matters as specific programs or level of staffing because of the wide variety of correctional facilities with their differences in administrative and political imperatives. Issues such as what level of care or range of treatment modalities are required in which particular setting for various levels of functional disability are left to the clinical and administrative judgment of the facility staff. While one can arrive at some estimate of the staffing level from the guidelines detailed below [in the Task Force report] (by formulating and weighing these requirements according to the size of the facility along with the mission of mental health services in question), the essential element is that the services provided meet the broad guidelines of adequate mental health care as set out herein. (p. 5)

With the understanding that every facility is unique, that mental health treatment teams can be made up of a variety of different mixes of the respective professions, and that different mental health professionals may be in greater or shorter supply in different geographic areas. Moreover, licensure varies from state to state, and while the Task Force does not seek to promote any one rigid staffing formula for all jails and prisons, nonetheless, it is important to note that something of a consensus has been reached among correctional mental health experts, as well as in prison and jail litigation, as to caseloads of psychiatrists of patients receiving psychotropic medications. Because of the unique importance of psychotropic medications, and the unique role of psychiatry in providing such medications, it is imperative that every system have enough psychiatrists to provide these services.

To begin, it must be appreciated that jails are much more diverse than prisons, and thus their staffing needs will vary. It is suggested that in jails, for every 75–100 inmates with serious mental illnesses who are receiving psychotropic medication, there be one full-time psychiatrist or equivalent. In prisons, with fewer admissions, the caseload of each full-time psychiatrist or equivalent can rise to a maximum of 150 patients on psychotropic medication.

Nevertheless, the Task Force just as clearly believes that adequate numbers of appropriately trained staff, in a variety of mental health professions, performing duties for which they are trained and authorized, must be present in every jail and prison. Staffing must be adequate to ensure that every inmate with serious mental illness or in psychiatric or emotional crisis has timely access to evaluation by a competent mental health professional. More important than the number of staff is *access* to adequate care.

IV. Education and Training

Professional development for mental health clinicians working in a jail or prison is essential. Participation of each practitioner in the educational and training program of the facility, as well as in other continuing medical education activities, is of great benefit to the facility as well as to each practitioner.

The educational and training program of the facility should include substantial "cross training," of security staff by clinical staff and vice versa. Mental health professionals will benefit from training and orientation by security staff to the jail or prison "culture," to include such matters as social order, gang affiliations, and attitudes toward sexual offenders, as well as utilization and/or manipulation of the mental health practitioner and system.

The work in a correctional setting may be frustrating and exhausting. By setting aside specific times for teaching and supervision, practitioners may be able to minimize "burnout" and, at the same time, fulfill a basic responsibility. Similarly, the employment agreement with the facility or system should provide specifically for such activities.

Ideally, each practitioner should receive specialty education and training at various levels prior to undertaking employment in a correctional setting. Education and training in correctional psychiatry should be available in medical schools and psychiatric residencies. Facilities should seek expertise in special applications described in this report through various means, such as recruitment of staff with subspecialty training, continuing professional education, and consultation. Each correctional psychiatrist should seek out relevant courses as continuing professional education or, at a minimum, the literature that is found in textbooks and journals.

Practitioners should communicate with colleagues who are working in other correctional facilities to share experiences and provide mutual support. In addition, practitioners are advised to become familiar with and consider joining subspecialty organizations, such as the American Academy of Psychiatry and the Law, which provide for continuing education and subgroups that share this interest. There are several other organizations of interest, including the American Correctional Health Services Association and the National Commission on Correctional Health Care. It should be noted that the Accreditation Council on Graduate Medical Education requires that fellowship programs for certification in forensic psychiatry include a substantial component in correctional expertise.

Because of the high prevalence of substance abuse among mentally ill offenders and its impact on the treatment of mental illness, expertise in substance abuse treatment is an important component of any correctional mental health system. This expertise may be provided by a psychiatrist or other mental health professional or an individual trained in an organized program of education and training in substance abuse recognition, prevention, and treatment.

Each psychiatrist prescribing medication for any inmate with substance abuse problems should have education, training, and/or consultation in substance abuse and the treatment of co-occurring (mental illness and substance abuse) disorders.

Similarly, several conditions are more frequently encountered in correctional settings than in the general practice of psychiatry. Examples include psychopathy, sexual disorders, and malingering. The ability to detect malingering is especially important, because although the mere presence of malingering does not preclude a finding of mental illness, as a rule malingerers can be wasteful of resources and therefore detract from the quality of services that psychiatrists can provide to patients who are truly in need of treatment.

Each psychiatrist practicing in a correctional setting should participate in the development of programs for teaching mental health principles to other professionals in the facility. Similarly, the participation of each practitioner in the ongoing educational program of the facility is good medical practice. In a correctional setting, custodial professionals and mental health (and other medical) professionals benefit from cross-professional training by participating in the others' in-service training.

An active liaison and/or affiliation with an academic-medical or other educational institution(s) is advantageous in recruitment, retention, continuing education, career satisfaction, and achievement and maintenance of high-quality services.

V. Cultural Awareness

A number of factors make the need for training in cultural diversity particularly important in correctional facilities. Jail and prison populations include high percentages of individuals from minority ethnic groups, and this contributes to cultural differences between the correctional staff, including mental health staff, and the inmates. Another cultural difference may arise from the fact that many correctional psychiatrists grew up and trained in countries other than the United States.

In order to properly evaluate and treat inmates in a correctional setting, it is imperative that clinicians and staff overcome the consequences of these often substantial cultural differences in background, socioeconomic class, education, and other types of diversities. Correctional facilities should provide training to ensure sensitivity to such cultural differences and support efforts to overcome the negative consequences of the cultural diversity, especially those that adversely affect the delivery of mental health services.

Such training should seek to ensure positive attitudes and acceptance of other cultures by means of didactic and experiential components. The goals and objects of such training should relate to attitude, knowledge, and skills. It is known that positive attitudes and acceptance of other cultures is often a learned phenomenon based on exposure to and awareness of other belief systems. Attitude changes that should be sought include improved tolerance of diverse populations, empathy for the minority experience (including the internalization of experiences of prejudice), and an understanding of concepts of ethnocentric bias and its potential effects.

The general overview of the program should contain information common to minority and ethnic groups and information about the specific ethnic groups with which an individual clinician will most often interface. Some themes to be pursued might include demographic information and epidemiology, the psychological aspects of immigration, the psychological aspects of minority status, religious and other beliefs and attitudes about psychiatric treatments, and sources of misdiagnosis and frequently misdiagnosed problems.

The didactic curriculum should include the presentation of biological, psychological, sociological, economic, ethnic, gender, religious/spiritual, sexual orientation, and family factors that significantly influence physical and psychological development.

Finally, the clinical training of correctional personnel should provide instruction about American culture and subcultures, particularly those found in the patient community associated with the facility.

VI. Informed Consent

Respect for the individual is a core value of the practice of medicine and psychiatry. Obtaining the consent of each patient is a reflection of that respect. The issue of consent poses special problems throughout the practice of psychiatry because the competency of an individual may be in question and/or because some emergency exists. The inherently coercive settings of lockups, jails, and prisons create additional difficulties.

The principles of informed consent as embodied in the ethical guidelines of the APA, the APA's *The Principles of Medical Ethics With Annotations Especially Applicable to Psychiatry*, based on the American Medical Association's *Principles of Medical Ethics*, remain applicable to patients in lockups, jails, and prisons. The patient should participate, to the extent possible, in decisions about evaluation and treatment. Psychiatrists should offer to discuss with their patients the nature, purpose, risks, and benefits of the potential types of treatment. Policies concerning the right to refuse treatment should conform with the rules and procedures of the jurisdiction in which the facility is located.

VII. Confidentiality

With recognition of the inevitable and, indeed, necessary loss of privacy in lockups, jails, and prisons, the usual principles of psychiatric confidentiality as embodied in the ethical guidelines of the APA, the APA's *The Principles of Medical Ethics With Annotations Especially Applicable to Psychiatry*, based on the American Medical Association's *Principles of Medical Ethics*, should, nevertheless, apply in all aspects of the delivery of psychiatric services. However, the special requirements presented by these settings, especially in relation to security, necessitate certain modifications. These modifications are grounded in the duties and responsibilities of custody staff as well as the safety and security of patients, other inmates, and staff. On the other hand, confidentiality may be particularly important to groups that are frequently encountered in correctional settings. Thus, the lack of privacy may have serious consequences for persons with HIV/AIDS, persons who have experienced sexual violence, sex offenders, and so forth.

In all situations, the rights of the patient to privacy and confidentiality must be weighed against the needs of other inmates as well as the institutional needs of safety and security. A distinction must be drawn between information obtained by a mental health professional in the course of treatment and information obtained from the inmate in the course of a forensic or other evaluation for nontreatment purposes. Some examples of the latter types of examinations are an evaluation, at the request of a court, for an evaluation of competency to stand trial or criminal responsibility, or a report for the parole board. More complex ethical issues are raised when a treating psychiatrist is asked to determine whether a patient can be sanctioned for an infraction or rules violation. In these cases, the usual rules in regard to confidentiality typically do not apply. It is the responsibility of the evaluating psychiatrist to set forth clearly to the inmate any such limitations on confidentiality as part of the informed consent process.

Similarly, in a treatment situation, mental health professionals must clearly specify any limits on the usual precepts of confidentiality prior to initiating treatment, except in emergencies. This notice may be presented in general terms, as applying to situations in which the patient or the institution may be at risk.

Some treatment situations in which the usual rules of confidentiality may not be applicable are

a. When the patient is self-injurious or suicidal.
b. When the patient is assaultive or homicidal.
c. When the patient presents a clear and present risk of escape or the creation of disorder within the facility.

This list is not meant to be all-inclusive and may be supplemented in accordance with the special needs of each patient or the institution. Additionally, certain situations in a jail or prison that are part of the mental health treatment process may require changes from the usual rules of confidentiality. Such situations may include when a patient is receiving psychotropic medication; when a patient requires movement to a special unit for observation, evaluation, or treatment of an acute episode; or when a patient requires transfer to a treatment facility outside the lockup, jail, or prison.

Whatever the limitations being placed on the usual rules of confidentiality, as expressed in the various laws and codes of ethics that apply, those rules, in general, should prevail. The exceptions relate to the legal, ethical, and moral obligations of staff to respond to dangerousness and the issues of internal disorder and escape.

Mental health professionals must be able to acquire patients' historical medical and mental health records from places where they have received previous services, within or outside of the correctional system, and ensure that records developed within the system move between facilities.

Mental health care professionals should share relevant confidential information with facility administrators (on a "need to know" basis) when it relates to the medical management of a patient, security issues, or a patient's ability to participate in programs.

As regards both evaluation and treatment, it is important that the mental health professional consider

   a. the role conflict in seeking to balance the therapeutic needs of the patient vis-à-vis the security and stability of the institution.
   b. the problems inherent in accurately predicting violence and dangerousness.
   c. the impact of any breach of confidentiality on the relationship with the inmate.

Mental health professionals should be able to communicate relevant confidential information to community providers when the patient is discharged.

In light of these special considerations, it is particularly important that specific, written policies be developed and maintained in regard to issues relating to confidentiality. In facilities where no written policy exists, it is the responsibility of the psychiatrist to clarify these issues with the institutional authorities and to develop working policies as to the degree to which confidentiality of information can be ensured.

Finally, these policies regarding confidentiality in lockups, jails, and prisons must be presented to, and discussed with, both staff and inmates. Provisions for this education and disclosure should be included in the facility's manual of operations.

VIII. Suicide Prevention

The risk of suicide is higher among incarcerated jail and prison inmates than among the population at large. An increased risk of suicide associated with mental illness also has been found. For these reasons, it is universally understood and legally required that each jail and prison have a suicide prevention program for identifying and responding to each suicidal inmate.

It is important to emphasize that an inmate may become suicidal at any point during his or her incarceration. High-risk periods include the time immediately upon admission to a lockup, jail, or prison; following new legal problems (e.g., new charges, additional sentences, institutional proceedings, denial of parole); following the receipt of bad news regarding one's self or one's family (e.g., a serious illness in the family or the loss of a loved one); and after suffering some type of humiliation (e.g., sexual assault) or rejection (e.g., by a significant other or child or loved one). An inmate who is placed in and is unable to cope with administrative segregation or other specialized single-cell housing assignment may also be at increased risk of suicide. An inmate who is in the early stages of recovery from severe depression is very much at risk, as well.

An adequate suicide prevention program must include the following components:

- Training of all staff who interact directly with inmates in how to recognize danger signs and what to do when they believe that an inmate may be suicidal
- Identification, through admission screening and referral, of inmates at heightened risk of suicide
- Policies to ensure adequate monitoring of suicidal inmates to prevent the loss of life
- Effective and well-understood referral system that allows staff and inmates to bring a suicidal inmate to the prompt attention of mental health staff

- Timely evaluation by mental health clinicians to determine the level of risk posed by an inmate who has been referred by screening or correctional staff
- Housing options that allow for adequate monitoring of suicidal inmates by staff
- Communication between mental health, correctional, medical, and other staff of the specific needs and risks presented by a suicidal inmate
- Timely provision of mental health services, including medication, verbal therapies, and crisis intervention, for chronically or acutely suicidal inmates
- Accurate and behaviorally specific reports documenting behaviors or statements that indicate suicide risk
- Review of incidents of suicide attempts or completed suicides, to improve institutional practices and to prevent unnecessary future occurrences
- Critical incident debriefing in the event of a completed suicide, to assist staff and inmates in dealing with predictable feelings of guilt, fear, grief, and anger

IX. Mental Health Treatment

Constitutional and statutory law, as well as these guidelines, requires that an inmate in a correctional setting have access to mental health treatment. This section of the principles governing the delivery of psychiatric services in jails and prisons seeks to clarify the purposes of such treatment and the modalities that may be employed.

Timely and effective access to mental health treatment is the hallmark of adequate mental health care. The principles and guidelines for psychiatric services in jails and prisons outlined in this document seek to ensure such access by setting out the parameters of access in the form of appropriate screening, referral, and mental health evaluation and treatment.

Mental health treatment in the correctional setting, like that in any setting, is defined as the use of a variety of mental health therapies, including biological, psychological, and social. In the correctional setting the goal of treatment is to alleviate symptoms of mental disorders that significantly interfere with an inmate's ability to function in the particular criminal justice environment in which the inmate is located. It is obvious, therefore, that mental health treatment is more than mere prescribing of psychotropic medication, and psychiatrists should resist being limited to this role.

The fundamental policy goal for correctional mental health treatment is to provide the same level of mental health services to each patient in the criminal justice process that should be available in the community. The purposes of mental health treatment in jails and prisons include 1) enabling patients to avail themselves of the rights of due process; 2) making the correctional facility safer for everyone who lives, works, or visits there; 3) relieving the unnecessary extremes of human suffering; and 4) permitting inmates the opportunity to make use of programs offered.

Thus, at the level of the lockup, the purposes of mental health treatment include benefits to the detainee's health and safety, with the outcome of restored competency to be arraigned. In a pretrial setting, the treatment might have the outcome of the restoration of competency to stand trial. In a prison setting, the outcome might be to return the inmate to the general population with the ability to participate in prison programs, including suitable mental health programs, and preparation for release.

Program priorities include, but are not limited to, the following:

- Recognizing and providing access to treatment for each inmate with serious mental illness or in psychiatric crisis
- Consulting with other health care providers and correctional administrators and staff
- As resources permit, treating patients who are in need of mental health care but who are not seriously and persistently mentally ill or in acute psychiatric crisis

Mental health treatment can occur in a number of different settings, including

- Acute care program
- Longer-term program
- Transitional care program
- Outpatient treatment program
- Inpatient hospital treatment program

Treatment modalities should be provided in a way that is consistent with generally accepted psychiatric practices and with institutional requirements.

A. Referral for Mental Health Treatment

Referral is the process by which an individual in the criminal justice process—having been identified through reception screening, mental health intake screening, or various processes at any time thereafter (including self-referral) as possibly in need of mental health treatment—is provided with the opportunity for a suitable mental health evaluation so that it can be determined whether such care is necessary.

The referral process may be simple or complex, depending on the facility, the urgency of the situation, and the mental health coverage provided. In each case, the referral process should be specifically defined and the roles of the various participants clearly delineated.

Referrals should be time constrained—that is, a maximum time for response to each referral, suitable to the situation, should be set out in the facility's operating standards. Timely referral and response should be designated as indicators of quality care.

B. Mental Health Evaluations

The nature and quality of the particular mental health evaluation are related to its context. In a lockup, where the major focus may be the removal of an inmate with severe mental illness to a psychiatric facility, evaluations tend to be brief and focused. In a jail or prison, where various levels of mental health housing and treatment may be available, such evaluations and interventions may be more detailed and extensive.

C. Therapeutic Milieu

To the extent possible, treatment should be provided in a setting that is conducive to the achievement of its goals. This includes not only the physical setting but also the social-emotional setting, in which an atmosphere of empathy and respect for the dignity of the patient is maintained.

A therapeutic milieu implies the following conditions:

- A sanitary and humane environment
- Written procedures and adequate staffing to permit adequate observation
- Adequate allocation of resources for the prevention of suicide and assault
- Medical and mental health staff available to provide adequate treatment and supervision
- Social interactions that foster recovery
- Transfer to an appropriate mental health facility according to a written policy approved by the mental health authority and the correctional facility administration when these conditions are not able to be met

As safety and security allow, self-help and peer support programs or activities contribute to the overall goals of the mental health services and should be promoted and encouraged by the clinical professional staff.

D. Discharge Planning

Timely and effective discharge planning is essential to continuity of care and an integral part of adequate mental health treatment. This is true whether the patient is being released into the community or transferred to another correctional facility. Because discharges (e.g., from jails) or transfers (e.g., between prisons) may occur on short notice, it is recommended that discharge planning be a part of the initial treatment plan. Appropriate communication with security staff, especially in cases of a short length of stay, would be facilitated by an adequate Management Information System.

Confidentiality concerns should be addressed to facilitate sharing of information among providers in different settings.

The essential services that are included in adequate discharge planning in jails and in prisons are listed in Part 2 of these guidelines. These include assessments, appointments to be arranged, notifications, staff responsibilities, linkages to community-based services, and so forth.

In addition, adequate discharge planning may include help with the obtaining of necessary financial benefits (e.g., Medicaid) and housing (because of the high incidence of homelessness in the jail and prison populations), placements, and appropriate linkages. Adequate discharge planning should also take into account the benefits of the assertive community therapy model for persons requiring a very structured and comprehensive discharge plan.

Finally, the important potential role of the family, when available, should be included in the discharge planning process.

X. Ethical Issues

Issues relating to ethics are of particular concern to psychiatrists practicing in correctional facilities because of the inherently coercive environment of jails and prisons and the pervasiveness of complex problems of dual loyalty.

The term *dual loyalty* is used to describe those situations in which a psychiatrist is subject to more than one authority or perhaps more than one moral principle. This problem, which also has been described as the "double agent problem," is unmistakable when a psychiatrist is working in a correctional facility. In this setting the conflict is between two distinct roles and responsibilities for the psychiatrist: his or her role and responsibilities as the inmate's treating physician versus his or her role and responsibilities as an employee or agent of the facility—that is, a local or state correctional agency or a company or an institution that staffs or operates the correctional facility, or perhaps more than one of these.

Conflicts in orientation, mission, purpose, aims, objectives, and even value systems arise from the psychiatrist's duties to the patient clashing with his or her duties to the department of correction or other organization or institution that are, in a way, his or her duties to "society." Correctional psychiatrists must be aware of these conflicts that may underlie their choices and decisions.

These concerns are heightened by the additional fact that psychiatrists practicing in criminal justice settings not only treat patients who are involved in the criminal justice system but also, as a separate and distinct function, may carry out psychiatric *evaluations* for legal purposes (e.g., evaluations of competency to stand trial, or, in a prison, reporting to a parole board). The importance of this distinction—between treatment and evaluation—is that the professional responsibilities that govern these roles—that is, the ethical principles that guide the psychiatrist in each situation—are dramatically different and are quite distinct in one role as contrasted to the other. Briefly, while the *treatment* responsibilities of the correctional psychiatrist may, overall, be governed by the usual principles of medical ethics—the principles of beneficence and nonmalfeasance (for the benefit of the patient and "do no harm")—the *evaluation* responsibilities of the forensic psychiatrist to the legal system are governed by very different principles—those of justice and the search for truth.

A model of separating these two separate and distinct roles and responsibilities is the accreditation standard of the National Commission on Correctional Health Care that explicitly prohibits health care workers from collecting "forensic information." The standard on "Forensic Information" in the *Standards for Health Services in Prisons* of the National Commission on Correctional Health Care (1997) requires that "written policy and procedures prohibit the prison's health care personnel from participating in the collection of certain information for forensic purposes." In its discussion of this standard, the commission elaborates on the differences between treating patients and acting in "forensic" matters by noting that

> [t]he role of the health care staff is to serve the health needs of inmate-patients. The position of its members as neutral, caring health care professionals is compromised when they are asked to collect information about inmates that may be used against the latter. Performing psychological evaluation of inmates for use in adversarial proceedings [is an example] of inappropriate uses of a facility's health care staff. Such acts undermine the credibility of these professionals with their patients, and compromise them by asking them to participate in acts that are usually done without inmates' consent.

However, the National Commission adds that where there is the problem that "state laws and regulations require that such acts [i.e., collecting "forensic information"] be performed by health care professionals, including mental health staff," then "the services of outside providers or someone on the institution's staff who is not involved in a therapeutic relationship with the inmate should be obtained."

This concept of recruiting a different member of the health care staff (i.e., one who is not in a treatment relationship with the particular patient) is a model that should be used in situations where the correctional psychiatrist is called on to perform responsibilities other than treating the patient. Thus, for example, psychiatrists practicing in some state prisons may be called on, or perhaps required, to provide information to a parole board. To avoid ethical conflicts, it is recommended that an effort be made to have such information obtained and provided to the parole board by a psychiatrist other than the treating psychiatrist. The general principle is that, where possible, the treating psychiatrist should seek to have another professional, who is not in a treating relationship with the patient, perform the "forensic responsibility" as is suggested by the standards of the National Commission on Correctional Health Care noted above.

In the introduction to the first edition of these guidelines (1989), it was noted that "the psychiatrist practicing in these settings is *always* bound by the standards of professional ethics as set out in the APA's Annotations Especially Applicable to Psychiatry to the AMA's Principles of Medical Ethics. These are the most fundamental statements of the moral and ethical foundations of professional psychiatric practice" (p. 5).

However, only two of the APA annotations specifically apply to psychiatrists practicing in a criminal justice setting. The first annotation relates to a period of time very early in the criminal justice process: before an individual has been arraigned. Annotation 13 to Section 4 of the *Principles of Medical Ethics With Annotations Especially for Psychiatry* states that "ethical considerations in medical practice preclude the psychiatric *evaluation* of any person charged with criminal acts prior to access to, or availability of, legal counsel. The only exception is the rendering of care to the person for the sole purpose of medical *treatment*" (emphasis added).

It is significant to note that here too, at the very beginning of the legal process—even before the arraignment process—there is a distinction made between a treating responsibility and an evaluation obligation. The point is that before a person who has been arrested has been before a judge (and usually has not spoken to a lawyer and been informed of the charges and apprised of his or her rights), a forensic psychiatric *evaluation* should not be performed.

Interestingly, the only other annotation relating to correctional psychiatry relates to a time at the end of the criminal justice process: when the inmate is to be executed. Annotation 4 of Section 1 of the *Principles of Medical Ethics With Annotations Especially for Psychiatry* states that "a psychiatrist should not be a participant in a legally authorized execution." Here, too, it seems that a distinction is being drawn between the psychiatrist's responsibility to treat the inmate (and the responsibility to benefit the patient) and a duty or responsibility to the state.

In this regard, the National Commission's approach—to use "the services of outside providers" (but *not*, in the case of executions, "someone on the institution's staff who is not involved in a therapeutic relationship with the inmate")—is set forth in a position statement of the commission (National Commission on Correctional Health Care 1988), titled on "Competency for Execution." It is stated that

> [t]he National Commission on Correctional Health Care's standards require that the determination of whether an inmate is "competent for execution" should be made by an independent expert and not by any health care professional regularly in the employ of, or under contract to provide health care with, the correctional institution or system holding the inmate. This requirement does not diminish the responsibility of correctional health care personnel to treat any mental illness of death row inmates.

The American Academy of Psychiatry and the Law has addressed matters relating to correctional psychiatry in more detail. Under the heading of confidentiality, *The Ethics Guidelines for the Practice of Forensic Psychiatry* of the American Academy of Psychiatry and the Law (1991) state that

> in a *treatment* situation, whether in regard to an inpatient or to an outpatient in a parole, probation, or conditional release situation, the psychiatrist should be clear about any limitations on the usual principles of confidentiality in the *treatment* relationship and assure that these limitations are communicated to the patient. The psychiatrist should be familiar with the institutional policies in regard to confidentiality. Where no policy exists, the psychiatrist should clarify these matters with the institutional authorities and develop working guidelines to define his role. (emphasis added)

As regards consent, *The Ethics Guidelines for the Practice of Forensic Psychiatry* of the American Academy of Psychiatry and the Law (1991) state that

> [c]onsent to *treatment* in a jail or prison or other criminal justice setting must be differentiated from consent to *evaluation*. The psychiatrists providing treatment in these settings should be familiar with the jurisdiction's rules in regard to the patient's right to refuse treatment. (emphasis added)

Then, more broadly, the guidelines state:

A *treating* psychiatrist should generally avoid agreeing to be an expert witness or to perform an *evaluation of his patient for legal purposes* because a *forensic evaluation* usually requires that other people be interviewed and testimony may adversely affect the therapeutic relationship. (emphasis added)

Here too, a clear distinction is made between treatment and evaluation.

Finally, we note that there is one code of ethics that seeks to apply ethical principles specifically to clinical practice in correctional settings: that of the American Correctional Health Services Association (ACHSA). The Preamble of the ACHSA Code of Ethics (1990) notes that

[t]he ACHSA code of ethics does not emerge in a vacuum. There are the codes of ethics of the professional disciplines. There are also international principles of law and ethics, such as the World Medical Association Declaration of Tokyo, the United Nations Principles of Medical Ethics, the United Nations Standard Minimum Rules for the Treatment of Prisoners and the International Council of Nurses Statement of the Role of the Nurse in Care of Detainees and Prisoners.

The ACHSA Code of Ethics goes on to specify that the correctional health professional should

Evaluate the inmate as a patient or client in each and every health care encounter.

Render medical treatment only when it is justified by an accepted medical diagnosis. Treatment and invasive procedures shall be rendered after informed consent.

Afford inmates the right to refuse care and treatment. Involuntary treatment shall be reserved for emergency situations in which there is grave disability and immediate threat of danger to the inmate or others.

Provide sound privacy during health services in all cases and sight privacy whenever possible.

Provide health care to all inmates regardless of custody status.

Identify themselves to their patients and not represent themselves as other than their professional license or certification permits.

Collect and analyze specimens only for diagnostic testing based on sound medical principles.

Perform body cavity searches only after training in proper techniques and when they are not in a patient-provider relationship with the inmate.

Not be involved in any aspect of execution of the death penalty.

Ensure that all medical information is confidential and health care records are maintained and transported in a confidential manner.

Honor custody functions but not participate in such activities as escorting inmates, forced transfers, security supervision, strip searches or witnessing use of force.

Undertake biomedical research on prisoners only when the research methods meet all requirements for experimentation on human subjects and individual prisoners or prison populations are expected to derive benefits form the results of the research.

Thus, while the ACHSA Code of Ethics does not explicitly distinguish between treatment and evaluation functions, this distinction is implicit in three separate sections: 1) collecting and analyzing specimens only for diagnostic purposes—presumably for treatment purposes; 2) body cavity searches, which should be performed only "when [the correctional health professional is] not in a patient-provider relationship with the inmate"; and, in the same spirit, 3) the injunction to honor "custody functions but not participate in such activities as escorting inmates, forced transfers, security supervision, strip searches or witnessing use of force."

Finally, we wish to repeat and emphasize the statement that appeared in the introduction to the first edition of these guidelines (1989):

[T]he psychiatrist practicing in these settings is always bound by the standards of professional ethics as set out in the APA's Annotations Especially Applicable to Psychiatry to the AMA's Principles of Medical Ethics. These are the most fundamental statements of the moral and ethical foundations of professional psychiatric practice.

XI. Research

Research is the basis upon which providing quality care to patients is developed. Psychiatric research may contribute to the community at large by investigating methods to improve public safety. Psychiatric research may assist mental health practitioners in their clinical work and help inmate patients. However, research with prisoners as subjects requires special legal safeguards and clinical considerations.

In addition to precautions accorded to each patient in studies, researchers must provide extra safeguards pertaining to the subjects' incarceration, in that the incarceration itself may be viewed as an inherently coercive setting that undermines an inmate's ability to provide freely given informed consent for participation in research.

The guidelines set forth in the Federal Regulations on Medical Research in Correctional Institutions by the Department of Health and Human Services (45 Code of Federal Regulation [CFR] 46, revised as of October 1, 1994) should be strictly observed, and all pharmacological research must comply with U.S. Food and Drug Administration (FDA) regulations that control the conduct of drug trials with prison populations.

Other types of research design, including epidemiological and noninvasive studies, can yield useful information about the precursors of mental illness in offenders, incidence and prevalence of mental illness, program design, physical plant design, and planning for services. However, the many complex issues in regard to research in these settings are beyond the scope of these guidelines.

XII. Administration and Administrative Issues

The effective provision of access to mental health services in correctional settings requires that there be a balance between security and treatment needs. It remains the conclusion of the APA that there is no fundamental incompatibility between good security and good treatment. It should be universally recognized that good treatment can contribute to good security and good security can contribute to good treatment.

The effective provision of mental health services requires that the mental health services administration be integrated into the overall management of the facility. Indeed, a comprehensive treatment program requires the close integration of clinical and security services. Furthermore, within clinical services, it is imperative that mental health services—psychiatric and psychological—be integrated with medical and substance abuse services.

A qualified health care administrator with a sound clinical background should have supervisory authority over the various professionals who work with mental health patients. This should include at least some specified authority over security staff on specialized mental health units.

Mental health administrative personnel in a jail or prison should establish written policies on critical issues such as staffing patterns, admission, referral, discharge criteria, health care management, information management, and interagency and intraagency communications, especially as regards confidential medical and mental health information.

The psychiatrist should take a leadership role in administrative as well as clinical issues. Even when control may be in the hands of nonpsychiatrists, attention always must be focused on the priorities of quality care and the best interests of the patient.

Each mental health professional should have training in and understanding of security needs and issues.

An environment that promotes therapeutic interactions may be created in a jail or a prison setting if there is clinical leadership with authority, staffing, and resources to work toward such an environment. In addition, there should be a good working relationship between all disciplines, including nurses, psychologists, psychiatrists, social workers, correctional officers, and correctional counselors. Such a relationship is best accomplished when a mental health administrator, who has clinical experience, serves as the coordinator among the different mental health disciplines.

It is especially important to have clinical input when decisions are made about an inmate who is receiving mental health care regarding disciplinary issues, work and housing assignments, and transfers in and out of the institution. For example, it is often important, clinically, for an inmate to be held accountable for his or her actions when the behavior is *not* a product of mental illness. Good communication between mental health and correctional professionals is essential if they are to effectively respond to manipulative behavior and to provide inmates with positive ways to meet their legitimate needs.

Each mental health professional working in a correctional setting should work within his or her own profession's scope of practice, as defined in that jurisdiction's licensure process (usually by the state), and within his or her own training, expertise, and skills. As such, mental health professionals provide services within a standard of care. However, chronic shortage of professional resources is a common problem in correctional settings. Although circumstances might engender a "siege mentality," one should not compromise professional responsibility. At the very least, a psychiatrist's responsibility includes communicating shortcomings and resource needs to the appropriate authority.

Mental health staff should be informed about and sensitive to the concerns of security staff. The relevant body of information regarding security should be mastered by mental health professionals as part of the education and training for working in these settings. Similarly, an organized program should be developed to teach and train correctional personnel about mental health issues. Among the programs that will especially benefit from carefully administered integration are those relating to developmental disabilities, neurological impairments, alcohol and drug abuse, and sex offenses.

XIII. Interprofessional Relationships

The adequate delivery of mental health services in jails and prisons requires the cooperation of all participating professionals, including psychiatrists, psychologists, social workers, nurses and other health care staff, correctional counselors, and correctional officers. The manner in which these professionals interact is critical to providing adequate care.

However, effective mental health treatment can be provided only in a safe environment. Consistent with our principle that "the effective provision of access to mental health services in correctional settings requires that there be a balance between security and treatment needs," all mental health policy, procedures, and practices operate in the context that security and custody are the primary requirements of these institutions.

All mental health professionals working in jails and prisons should respect one another's particular expertise and contributions in order to work well together. In order for this to occur, mental health professionals of all disciplines need to be open with each other and free to consult with each other on a formal and informal basis. If this is done, areas of special skills can be established, which thereby creates an atmosphere of mutual confidence and trust.

Administrative supervision and clinical supervision of clinical staff require different types of expertise. In establishing supervisory relationships, it is recognized that in day-to-day responsibilities some administrative issues will impinge upon clinical decision making. Such issues include housing of inmates with mental illness and on-call coverage issues.

Many models of supervision are employed in correctional settings. Whatever model is utilized, it is important that the elements of the practical aspects of supervision be within the appropriate expertise of the supervisor. Whether mental health services are provided in a correctional setting by the psychiatric/mental health staff of the correctional department, by a separate department of mental health, or by private contractors, professional independence of clinical decisions should be maintained.

XIV. Psychiatric Services in Court and Other Settings

Care and treatment must be provided to each inmate regardless of the setting. Difficulties and crises may occur anywhere and at any time, including court trips and medical trips. Throughout the various stages of the criminal justice process, an individual may be brought from a particular facility to appear in court. Therefore, consideration must be given to providing psychiatric services in the court setting.

The stress that is usually attendant to a court appearance makes the court a locus of exacerbation. Clearly there must be some capacity for mental health consultation and crisis intervention. The court should consider having professionals available who can provide appropriate crisis intervention for persons with mental illness in the criminal justice process.

In addition, the court must be able to apply the mental health information it receives to the criminal justice process. For example, information regarding the presence of mental illness may be relevant to diversion of the defendant out of the criminal justice process itself. Similarly, professionals working in the court setting must have a means of transmitting the mental health information they receive to subsequent facilities and professionals who have a need to know such information.

It is the responsibility of the particular court and its administration to ensure that such services are established and available. However, in many cases, the provision of the services will be the responsibility of the facility or agency with then-current jurisdiction over the individual detainees, as when patients sent from jails or prisons are receiving medication during the course of their court appearance. (Arrangements for services to a patient in need of care and treatment are part of the transfer planning for the sending facility.)

XV. Jail Diversion and Alternatives to Incarceration

More than 500,000 persons with serious mental illnesses are admitted to U.S. jails each year. Many of these people could be kept out of or moved more quickly through the criminal justice process and out of jail if diversion programs were available. Mental health diversion programs transfer people from the criminal justice system to community-based mental health and substance abuse services. There are two types of diversion programs: prebooking and postbooking. *Prebooking* programs involve police and innovative emergency mental health responses that provide alternatives to booking mentally ill people into jail. *Postbooking* programs comprise three subtypes: 1) dismissal of charges in return for agreement for participation in a negotiated set of services, 2) deferred prosecution with requirements for treatment participation, and 3) post-sentence release in which conditions for probation include requirements for mental health and substance abuse services.

Some individuals with mental illnesses must be held in jail because of the seriousness of the offense they committed and/or their histories of nonappearance in court. They must have access to appropriate mental health treatment within the jail. However, many individuals with mental illnesses who have been arrested for less serious, nonviolent crimes should, where suitable, be diverted from jail to community-based mental health programs.

People who receive appropriate mental health treatment in the community usually have a better long-term prognosis and less chance of returning to jail for a similar offense than people who remain in jails without access to appropriate services. In addition, appropriate diversion of individuals with mental illnesses from the criminal justice system helps promote smooth jail operations.

The best diversion programs see detainees as citizens of the community who require a broad array of services, including mental health care, substance abuse treatment, housing, and social services. They recognize that some individuals come into contact with the criminal justice system as a result of fragmented services, the nature of their illnesses, and the lack of social support and other resources. They know that people should not be detained in jail simply because they are mentally ill. Only through diversion programs that address this fragmentation by integrating an array of mental health and other support services, including case management and housing, may the unproductive cycle of decompensation, disturbance, and arrest be broken.

PART 2

Guidelines for Psychiatric Services in Jails and Prisons

I. Introduction

The guidelines for psychiatric services in jails and prisons are based on the principles governing the delivery of psychiatric services presented in Part 1 of this document. In regard to the special populations of inmates with substance use disorders, inmates with co-occurring disorders, inmates with HIV/AIDS, women inmates, youth in adult correctional facilities, the geriatric population, and offenders with mental retardation or developmental disabilities, these guidelines are supplemented by the special applications of the principles and guidelines presented that will follow, in Part 3. It is important to reiterate that these guidelines are supplementary to the standards developed by the National Commission on Correctional Health Care.

The broad outline of these guidelines includes three basic types of services in jails and prisons: 1) screening, referral, and evaluation; 2) treatment; and 3) discharge planning.

II. Jails

A *jail* generally is defined as a detention or correctional facility where an individual is confined while awaiting trial or, in most jurisdictions, serving a sentence of 1 year or less. These facilities are usually under the jurisdiction of the county or municipality in which they are located. Jails are high-volume facilities. There are about 3,350 of these facilities around the country, processing approximately 10 million people each year.

There are great differences in the size of jails, ranging from a few cells to jails with thousands of inmates ("mega jails"). In larger jurisdictions, the jail is a system of correctional and detention facilities, each with different purposes and service needs. The specific policies and procedures for psychiatric services vary accordingly.

Confinement in a jail may occur for a variety of reasons. It also should be noted that in certain jurisdictions, the jail may be used to house people for civil charges, public health reasons, and detention for the Immigration and Naturalization Service, as well as serve as temporary housing for state and federal inmates. Each of these various purposes of confinement results in differing periods and conditions of confinement in the local jail.

Confinement in a jail usually takes place shortly after apprehension, and the stress level may be extremely high. Furthermore, conditions that may have prevailed at the time of the arrest, such as intoxication or psychosis, may still be acute. Acute symptoms of a mental disorder and/or a substance use disorder, acute intoxication, and the stressful conditions within a jail increase the risks of suicidal and violent behavior. Individuals with these conditions may have acute mental health needs that require an immediate response. In addition, a detainee may experience mental health problems or psychiatric crises during the course of the detention. Issues may arise concerning treatment, restraint and seclusion, safety of the staff and detainees, or emergency medical and psychiatric needs of detainees.

In jails, the core components of essential psychiatric services are screening and referral, assessment and evaluation, mental health treatment, and discharge planning.

A. Identification

1. Screening and Referral

a. Receiving Mental Health Screening and Referral

Definition
Receiving mental health screening is defined as mental health information and observations gathered for every newly admitted detainee during the intake procedures as part of the normal reception and classification process by using standard forms and following standard procedures. *Referral* is defined as the process by which inmates who appear to be in need of mental health treatment receive targeted assessment or evaluation so that they can be assigned to appropriate services.

Essential Services

1. Receiving mental health screening occurs immediately upon the detainee's arrival at the jail.
2. Receiving mental health screening consists of observation and structured inquiry into each detainee's mental health history and symptoms. Structured inquiry includes questions regarding suicide history, ideation, and potential; prior psychiatric hospitalizations and treatment; and current and past medications, both those prescribed and what is actually being taken.
3. Receiving mental health screening may be conducted by the booking officer and/or other custodial personnel, supervisor, etc., or by the medical intake nurse. Whoever provides this service must receive training in mental health screening and referral. Information about the detainee's behavior leading up to and during the arrest should be obtained from the arresting officer.
4. The purpose of receiving mental health screening is to determine whether the detainee, as a result of mental illness, may be dangerous to himself or herself or to others, or may be so acutely or seriously mentally ill that he or she requires immediate evaluation by a mental health professional or to be scheduled for a nonemergency mental health assessment or evaluation. The screening also should include recommendations for possible special care and custody. An acutely mentally ill or suicidal detainee should be transferred to a mental health treatment facility for stabilization or referred for immediate mental health evaluation and specialized housing or watched within the jail.
5. The receiving screening procedure and the questions asked should be standardized. Observations and responses should be documented on a standard form and made a part of the permanent health record.
6. Policies and procedures should specify what actions are required and within what time frames as a result of positive screening observations.
7. The psychiatrist may have a limited role in the direct provision of this service. The psychiatrist's three primary responsibilities are

   a. participating in the development of an appropriate screening form and screening procedures.
   b. training officers and health care personnel to use the screening

instrument and to make appropriate referrals.

c. working with facility officials to develop written referral procedures for inmates identified during the screening as being at high risk.

b. Intake Mental Health Screening and Referral

Definition

Intake mental health screening is defined as a more comprehensive examination performed on each newly admitted detainee within 14 days of arrival at an institution. It usually includes a review of the medical screening, behavioral observation, an inquiry into any mental health history, and an assessment of suicide potential. *Referral* is defined as the process by which detainees who appear to be in need of mental health treatment receive targeted assessment or evaluation so that they can be assigned to appropriate services.

Essential Services

1. Intake mental health screening should be conducted by a health care professional.
2. The intake mental health screening procedure and the questions asked should be standardized. Observations and responses should be documented and made a part of the permanent health record.
3. Policies and procedures should specify what actions are required and within what time frames as a result of positive screening observations.
4. At the time of the intake mental health screening, if no referral is necessary, detailed information regarding access to mental health services should be provided to the inmate.
5. The psychiatrist generally has a limited role in the direct provision of this service. The psychiatrist's four roles are

   a. participating in the development of appropriate intake mental health screening forms and informational material.
   b. training health care staff in the use of the intake mental health screening forms and the informational (orientation) materials.
   c. developing written referral procedures for inmates identified during the intake mental health screening process as requiring mental health evaluation.
   d. continuing or reviewing previously prescribed medication.

c. Postclassification Referral

Definition

During initial classification, information is gathered in order to assign inmates to appropriate housing and programs. Inmates who are not referred during either mental health screening process (receiving or intake) may subsequently demonstrate an apparent need for mental health services (including self-referral). *Postclassification referral* is defined as the process by which such individuals are brought to the attention of mental health staff for brief mental health assessment or comprehensive mental health evaluation.

Essential Services

1. The referral process may be simple or complex, depending on the facility, the urgency of the situation, and the mental health coverage provided. Specific written procedures providing for these types of referral should be part of the facility's mental health services plan.
2. Mental health emergency services must be accessible upon referral on a 24-hour basis.
3. An inmate awaiting mental health evaluation or transfer may require special precautions, including continuous observation, which should be maintained while the evaluation is pending.
4. Training of all health care and custody staff should be done on an ongoing basis and should include how and when to use the referral process.
5. All inmates must receive orientation and explanation of the operation of the referral process in a timely fashion.
6. The role of the psychiatrist in the referral process is to assist in the development of the policies and procedures for this activity and in training staff in the use of the referral system.

2. Brief Mental Health Assessment

Definition

A *brief mental health assessment* is defined as a mental health examination that is appropriate to the particular, suspected level of services needed and is focused on the suspected mental illness.

Essential Services

1. A brief mental health assessment should be conducted within 72 hours of the time of a positive screening and referral. In cases of urgency, provision should be made for immediate assessment evaluation upon referral. A brief mental health assessment should be completed for each individual whose screening reveals mental health problems in the procedures above, and a written recommendation should be prepared for any further evaluation and treatment, including possibly a comprehensive mental health evaluation (see next section). However, when it is clinically appropriate to do so, an individual may be referred directly for a comprehensive mental health evaluation without a brief mental health assessment.

2. The findings of the brief mental health assessment should be recorded on a standard form that is part of the confidential mental health record.

3. The brief mental health assessment should be conducted by an appropriately trained mental health professional.

4. The brief mental health assessment may or may not result in the development of a treatment plan.

5. The psychiatrist has both a direct and an indirect role in the provision of this service:

   a. The psychiatrist helps develop policies and procedures.
   b. The psychiatrist performs the mental health evaluation or consultation when appropriate and/or necessary. In some small jails, where a consulting psychiatrist may be the sole mental health practitioner, he or she will be a direct provider of this service.
   c. The psychiatrist may take responsibility for supervision of the mental health staff, administration of the mental health services, and liaison with other medical and administrative personnel in the facility.

3. Comprehensive Mental Health Evaluation

Definition

A comprehensive mental health evaluation consists of a face to face interview of the patient and a review of all reasonably available health care records and collateral information. It concludes with a diagnostic formulation and, at least, an initial treatment plan.

Essential Services

1. A comprehensive mental health evaluation may be indicated if treatment for a serious mental disorder at the jail facility is being contemplated and the brief mental health assessment is not adequate or appropriate, given its more focused content.
2. The comprehensive mental health evaluation should be conducted within a time frame appropriate to the level of urgency.
3. The findings of the comprehensive mental health evaluation should be recorded on a standard form that becomes part of the confidential mental health record.
4. The comprehensive mental health evaluation should be conducted by a psychiatrist or by another appropriately licensed or credentialed mental health professional.
5. The psychiatrist has both a direct and an indirect role in the provision of this service:

    a. The psychiatrist may perform all or part of the comprehensive mental health assessment when appropriate and/or necessary (e.g., when a detainee is already taking psychotropic medications).
    b. The psychiatrist may take responsibility for supervision of the mental health staff, administration of the mental health services, and liaison with other medical and administrative personnel in the facility.

6. The comprehensive mental health evaluation should include access to psychological and neuropsychological services.
7. The comprehensive mental health evaluation should include access to clinical laboratory and neuroimaging procedures.

B. Mental Health Treatment

Definition

The generic definition of *mental health treatment* has been given in Part 1 of this document. Considering the short-term nature of most jail confinements, treatment generally emphasizes crisis intervention, with prescribing of psychotropic medications and brief or supportive therapies and patient education. For the detainee whose pretrial confinement may be of longer term, more extensive verbal therapies and skill-building activities also may become part of the treatment regimen.

Essential Services

1. Inpatient resources either in jail (preferably licensed) or in an external hospital setting should be provided.
2. Seven-day-a-week mental health coverage (including coverage with a board-certified or board-eligible psychiatrist) should be provided.
3. A written treatment plan should be prepared for each inmate who is receiving ongoing mental health services.
4. A full range of psychotropic medications, including involuntary medication, must be available, with the capacity to administer them in an emergency.
5. Psychotropic medication should be prescribed and monitored by a psychiatrist.
6. Procedures should be developed and monitored by a psychiatrist to ensure that psychotropic medications are distributed by qualified medical personnel.
7. Seven-day-a-week, 24-hour nursing coverage must exist in any area where people with acute or emergent psychiatric problems are housed.
8. Special observation, seclusion, or restraint capability must exist.
9. Supportive and informative verbal interventions, in an individual or group context as clinically appropriate, should be provided.
10. Programs that provide productive, out-of-cell activity and teach necessary psychosocial and living skills should be provided.
11. All custodial staff must be trained in the recognition of mental disorders

C. Discharge Planning

Definition

Discharge planning in a jail setting is defined as all procedures through which each inmate in need of mental health care at the time of release from jail to the community or at the time of transfer to a prison is made known to the appropriate mental health service providers.

Essential Services

1. Appointments should be arranged with mental health agencies for all inmates with serious mental illness, especially those receiving psychotropic medication.

2. Reception centers at state prisons should be notified and/or arrangements should be made with local mental health agencies to have prescriptions renewed or evaluated for renewal and records shared as suitable.
3. The mental health treatment staff should ensure that discharge/referral responsibilities are carried out by specifically designated staff.
4. Each inmate to be released who has received mental health treatment services should be assessed for appropriateness of a community referral.
5. The prison classification/intake staff should be notified of the services received and the current clinical condition of every inmate transferred to prison who has received mental health crisis intervention or treatment services.
6. Jail mental health staff should participate in the development of any service contracts to ensure access to community-based case managers to provide continuity of services.

III. Prisons

A *prison* is generally defined as a correctional facility where an individual is confined to serve a sentence, usually in excess of 1 year. In contrast to jails, which are usually under the jurisdiction of the county or municipality in which they are located, prisons are operated by each state. The federal government also operates its own prison system, the Federal Bureau of Prisons. There are many fewer prisons than jails, and prisons usually house large numbers of inmates (more than 1,000 in most cases).

In contrast to detainees in lockups and jails, prison inmates often have been in the criminal justice system for an extended period of time. By the time an inmate arrives at prison, he or she often has been "in custody" for some time and faces mental health issues that frequently are different from those of an inmate who has just been arrested. However, because an increasing number of prison inmates in some jurisdictions are recently apprehended "parole violators," an increasing percentage of such inmates arrive at prison with mental health issues that are more commonly seen in those facing jail. Nonetheless, jail and prison inmate populations are likely to be somewhat different because of some general differences in these populations. For instance, the prison population, compared with the jail population, may have a lower incidence of more toxic or other acute psychotic states that may have been present at the time of the arrest or precipitated by the arrest and presumably have been the target of treatment. The prevalence of long-term psychotic illnesses in prison, however, is comparable to that in jail. By the time an inmate comes to prison, some psychological adaptation to the loss of liberty is more likely to have taken place. On the other hand, the stresses of being sentenced and transferred to a prison may create new pressures, such as separation stress due to a typically longer distance from family and friends, in addition to the stress of any transfer from one part of the correctional system to another.

Again, the components of essential mental health services in prisons are screening and referral, assessment and evaluation, mental health treatment, and discharge planning.

A. Identification

1. Screening and Referral

a. Receiving Mental Health Screening and Referral

Definition
Receiving mental health screening is defined as mental health information and observations gathered for every newly admitted inmate during the intake procedures as part of the normal reception and classification process by using standard forms and following standard procedures. *Referral* is defined as the process by which inmates who appear to be in need of mental health treatment receive targeted assessment or evaluation so that they can be assigned to appropriate services.

Essential Services

1. Receiving mental health screening occurs immediately upon the inmate's arrival at the prison.
2. Receiving mental health screening consists of observation of appearance and behavior and structured inquiry into the inmate's mental health history and symptoms. Structured inquiry includes questions regarding suicide history, ideation, and intention; prior treatment in jail; prior psychiatric hospitalizations; and current and past medications, both those prescribed and what is actually being taken.

3. Receiving mental health screening may be conducted by the receiving officer and/or other custodial personnel, classification officer, or supervisor, or by the medical intake nurse. Whoever provides this service must receive training in mental health screen-ing and referral.

4. The purpose of receiving mental health screening is to determine whether the inmate, as a result of mental illness, may be dangerous to himself or herself or to others, or may be so acutely or seriously mentally ill that he or she requires immediate evaluation by a mental health professional or to be scheduled for a nonemergency mental health assessment or evaluation. The screening also should include recommendations for possible special care and custody. An acutely mentally ill or suicidal inmate should be transferred to a mental health treatment facility for stabilization or referred for immediate mental health evaluation and specialized housing or watched within the prison.

5. The receiving mental health screening procedure and the questions asked should be standardized. Observations and responses should be documented and made a part of the permanent health record.

6. Policies and procedures should specify what actions are required and within what time frames as the result of positive screening observations.

7. The psychiatrist may have a limited role in the direct provision of this service. The psychiatrist's three primary roles in this regard are

    a. participating in the development of an appropriate screening form and screening procedures.
    b. training officers and health care personnel to use the screening instrument and to make appropriate referrals.
    c. working with facility officials to develop written referral procedures for inmates identified during the screening as being at high risk.

b. Intake Mental Health Screening and Referral

Definition

Intake mental health screening is defined as a more comprehensive examination performed on each newly admitted inmate within 14 days of arrival at an institution. It usually includes a review of the medical screening, behavioral observation, an inquiry into any mental health history, and an assessment of suicide potential. *Referral* is defined as the process by which inmates who appear to be in need of mental health treatment receive targeted assessment or evaluation so that they can be assigned to appropriate services.

Essential Services

1. Intake mental health screening should be conducted by a health care professional.
2. The intake mental health screening procedure and the questions asked should be standardized. Observations and responses should be documented and made a part of the permanent health record.
3. Policies and procedures should specify what actions are required and within what time frames as a result of positive screening observations.
4. At the time of the intake mental health screening, if no referral is necessary, detailed information regarding access to mental health services should be provided to the inmate.
5. The psychiatrist generally has a limited role in the direct provision of this service. The psychiatrist's four primary roles are

   a. participating in the development of the appropriate intake mental health screening forms and informational material.
   b. training health care staff in the use of the intake mental health screening forms and the informational (orientation) materials.
   c. working with facility officials to develop written referral procedures for inmates identified during the intake mental health screening process as requiring mental health evaluation.
   d. continuing or reviewing previously prescribed medication.

c. Postclassification Referral

Definition

During initial classification, information is gathered in order to assign inmates to appropriate housing and programs. Inmates who are not referred during either mental health screening process (receiving or intake) may subsequently demonstrate an apparent need for mental health services (including self-referral). *Postclassification referral* is defined as the process by which such individuals are brought to the attention of mental health staff for brief mental health assessment or comprehensive mental health evaluation.

Essential Services

1. The referral process may be simple or complex, depending on the facility, the urgency of the situation, and the mental health coverage provided. Specific written procedures providing for these types of referrals should be part of the facility's mental health services plan.
2. Mental health emergency services must be accessible on a 24-hour basis.
3. An inmate awaiting mental health evaluation or transfer may require special precautions, including continual observation, which should be maintained while the evaluation is pending.
4. Training of all health care and custody staff should be done on an ongoing basis and should include how and when to use the referral process.
5. All inmates must receive orientation and explanation of the operation of the referral process in a timely fashion.
6. The role of the psychiatrist in the referral process is to assist in the development of the policies and procedures for this activity and in training staff in the use of the referral system.

2. Brief Mental Health Assessment

Definitions

A *brief mental health assessment* is defined as a mental health examination that is appropriate to the particular, suspected level of services needed and is focused on the suspected mental illness.

Essential Services

1. A brief mental health assessment should be conducted within 72 hours of the time of a positive screening or referral. In cases of urgency, provision shall be made for immediate evaluation upon referral. A brief mental health assessment should be completed for the individual who is screened positively in the procedures above, and a written recommendation should be prepared for any further evaluation and treatment, including possibly a comprehensive mental health evaluation (see next section). However, when it is clinically appropriate to do so, an individual may be referred directly for a comprehensive mental health evaluation without a brief mental health assessment.

2. The findings of the brief mental health assessment should be recorded on a standard form that is part of the confidential mental health record.
3. The brief mental health assessment should be conducted by an appropriately trained mental health professional.
4. The brief mental health assessment may or may not result in the development of a treatment plan.
5. The psychiatrist has both a direct and an indirect role in the provision of this service:

    a. The psychiatrist develops policies and procedures.
    b. The psychiatrist performs the mental health evaluation or consultation when appropriate and/or necessary.
    c. The psychiatrist may take responsibility for supervision of the mental health staff, administration of the mental health services, and liaison with other medical and administrative personnel in the facility.

3. Comprehensive Mental Health Evaluation

Definition

A comprehensive mental health evaluation consists of a face-to-face interview of the patient and a review of all available health care records and collateral information. It concludes with a diagnostic formulation and, at least, an initial treatment plan.

Essential Services

1. A comprehensive mental health evaluation may be indicated if treatment for a serious mental disorder at the prison is being contemplated and the brief mental health assessment is not adequate or appropriate, given its more focused content.
2. The comprehensive mental health evaluation should be conducted within a time frame appropriate to the level of urgency.
3. The findings of the comprehensive mental health evaluation should be recorded in a standardized format that becomes part of the confidential mental health record.
4. The comprehensive mental health evaluation is conducted by a psychiatrist or by another appropriately licensed or credentialed mental health professional.

5. The psychiatrist has both a direct and an indirect role in the provision of this service:

    a. The psychiatrist may perform all or part of the comprehensive mental health assessment when appropriate and/or necessary (e.g., when an inmate is already taking psychotropic medications).

    b. The psychiatrist may take responsibility for supervision of the mental health staff, administration of the mental health services, and liaison with other medical and administrative personnel in the facility.

6. The comprehensive mental health evaluation should include access to psychological and neuropsychological services when indicated.

7. The comprehensive mental health evaluation should include access to clinical laboratory and neuroimaging procedures when indicated.

B. Mental Health Treatment

Definition

The generic definition of *mental health treatment* has been given in Part 1 of this document. It may include crisis intervention, including elements of suicide prevention (see section on suicide prevention in Part 1 of this document), and continuing treatment.

Essential Services

1. Inpatient resources either in prison (preferably licensed) or in an external hospital setting should be provided.

2. Seven-day-a-week mental health coverage (including coverage with a board-certified or board-eligible psychiatrist) should be provided.

3. A written treatment plan should be prepared for each inmate who is receiving ongoing mental health services.

4. A full range of psychotropic medications, including involuntary medication, must be available, with the capacity to administer them in an emergency.

5. Psychotropic medication should be prescribed and monitored by a psychiatrist.

6. Procedures should be developed and monitored by a psychiatrist to ensure that psychotropic medications are distributed by qualified medical personnel.
7. Seven-day-a-week, 24-hour nursing coverage must exist in any area where people with acute or emergent psychiatric problems are housed.
8. Special observation, seclusion, or restraint capability must exist.
9. Supportive and informative verbal interventions, in an individual or group context as clinically appropriate, should be provided.
10. Programs that provide productive, out-of-cell activity and teach necessary psychosocial and living skills should be provided.
11. All custodial staff must be trained in the recognition of mental disorders.

C. Discharge Planning

Definition

Discharge planning in a prison setting is defined as all procedures through which each inmate in need of mental health care at the time of release from prison is linked with appropriate community agencies capable of providing ongoing treatment, or at the time of transfer to a court or jail or another prison is made known to the appropriate mental health service providers in the court setting or jail or other prison.

Essential Services

1. Appointments should be arranged with mental health agencies for all inmates with serious mental illness, especially those receiving psychotropic medication.
2. Arrangements should be made with local mental health agencies to have prescriptions renewed or evaluated for renewal and records shared as suitable.
3. The mental health treatment staff should ensure that discharge/ referral responsibilities are carried out by specifically designated staff.
4. Each inmate to be released who has received mental health treatment services should be assessed for appropriateness of a community referral.
5. Prison administrative mental health staff should participate in the development of service contracts to ensure access to community-based case managers to provide continuity of services.

PART 3

Special Applications of the Principles and Guidelines

I. Introduction

There are particular population groups in jails and prisons whose evaluation and treatment are sufficiently unique as to warrant specific discussion to ensure an adequate level of care. These include inmates with substance use disorders, inmates with co-occurring disorders, inmates with HIV/AIDS, women inmates, youth in adult correctional facilities, the geriatric population (and the terminally ill population), and offenders with mental retardation or developmental disabilities. This section seeks to set out the special characteristics of each of these groups that must be considered to ensure their access to appropriate mental health services.

At the same time, it is important to acknowledge that there are other groups and conditions that are not addressed in these special applications. Future editions of these guidelines may undertake to assist in the development of special applications of these principles and guidelines to these groups and conditions. In the interim, psychiatrists should develop special clinical policies and procedures, as needed, for such groups and conditions.

The Task Force has not taken on the difficult issue of mental health services in juvenile correctional facilities. This is not to be taken as an indication that we believe this issue to be of lesser importance. To the contrary, it is precisely because of its importance that we suggest that an appropriate group, made up of experts in child and adolescent psychiatry, juvenile justice, and especially the treatment of serious mental illness and severe emotional disturbances among juvenile delinquents, be charged by the APA to undertake this effort.

II. Substance Use Disorders

Substance use disorder refers to substance abuse, substance dependence, intoxication, and withdrawal. Substance use disorder is the focus of the practice of addiction psychiatry. In the correctional setting, substance use disorder occurs with a high frequency, oftentimes with a co-occurring serious mental illness. The Task Force has chosen to cover substance use disorders and co-occurring disorders separately in these special applications of the principles and guidelines because they elicit separate clinical responses for psychiatric care.

It is estimated that up to 70%–90% of offenders may have a substance use disorder at the time of their entry into the criminal justice system. Criminal behavior often occurs when an individual is under the influence of alcohol or other drugs. Additionally, criminal behavior may be related to efforts to procure or sell the substance that is being abused. Indeed, much of the overall increase in the American prison population is ascribed to the alcohol and other drug use epidemic and changes in sentencing laws for these offenses.

While these requirements are especially important in receiving mental health screening in a jail setting, a substantial number of parole violators do enter prisons directly from the street. Therefore, services addressing substance use problems are highly relevant in both jails and prisons. Furthermore, even inmates who are being transferred between correctional facilities should not be presumed to be drug free.

An individual with a substance use disorder may present during receiving mental health screening with any of a variety of medical, neurological, or psychiatric problems. The receiving mental health screening instrument should include questions relating to the individual's use of alcohol and other drugs and the patterns of use, as well as observations related to whether or not the offender is presently under the influence of alcohol or drugs or experiencing withdrawal symptoms.

A positive receiving mental health screening for substance intoxication should trigger an immediate mental health screening for the presence of depressed mood and/or suicidal ideas. In a jail setting, most completed suicides occur within 24–48 hours after admission and are often carried out by inmates who are either intoxicated or experiencing withdrawal symptoms. Psychiatrists should have an important role in developing the receiving screening instrument, in training of staff in its use, and in educating correctional security, medical, and mental health staff about the signs and symptoms of intoxication and withdrawal.

Similarly, intake mental health screening should include questions in regard to an inmate's history of alcohol and other drug use as well as observations for the presence of signs of intoxication or withdrawal symptoms. Again, the role of the psychiatrist is in the development of the instrument and staff training.

The brief mental health assessment and the comprehensive mental health evaluation are particularly important in ensuring a proper diagnosis as the basis for the appropriate clinical management of an inmate with a substance use problem. When psychotropic medications are required during detoxification for management of medical or neurological symptoms, psychotic symptoms, or agitation, a physician, who may be a psychiatrist, should be responsible for managing the detoxification process.

The psychiatrist should develop a differential diagnosis as part of the comprehensive mental health evaluation to ensure that substance use disorders are recognized and that the sequelae of substance abuse are not misdiagnosed as major mental illness, and to consider the possibility of co-occurring substance abuse and mental disorders.

Prescription of benzodiazepines may be useful to prevent or attenuate withdrawal symptoms and detoxify the inmate. However, their use should be short term and on a tapering dosage schedule to ensure that the prescribed medication does not serve as a substitute for the substance of abuse. Other psychotropic medications should be prescribed judiciously for individuals with no prior history of mental illness. When circumstances warrant, an inmate should be detoxified or free of substance use for a reasonable period of time before psychotropic medications are prescribed unless psychotic or suicidal symptoms are present.

Substance abuse services should be integrated with mental health services. Psychosocial problems and skills deficiencies should be addressed with individualized programming, created through comprehensive assessment and consultation with the inmate's treatment provider, family (or significant other), and correctional medical and mental health clinicians.

Inmates with co-occurring mental illness should not be barred from participation in substance abuse treatment programs. Self-help, Twelve-Step, and peer support groups and networks play an important role in rehabilitation of alcohol and other drug abusers in the correctional system. Consideration should be given to allowing outside community support self-help meetings into the correctional setting to permit integration and identification with the community upon release.

Rehabilitation is a long-term commitment and must extend past the period of incarceration in order to have a positive impact on criminal recidivism and alcohol and other drug abstinence. Thus, discharge planning, when appropriate, should include referral to community-based substance abuse treatment.

III. Co-occurring Disorders

Co-occurring mental illness and substance use disorders often are undetected in people coming in contact with the justice system, because of the absence of effective screening and assessment and the difficulty in identifying the often complicated symptom picture with which this population presents.

Nondetection of one or more co-occurring disorders in the justice system may exacerbate behavior problems and elevate the risk of suicide and may result in poor outcomes in treatment during incarceration and rearrest and reincarceration after release. Combined with the stress and stigma associated with mental disabilities, the stress associated with arrest and charges may exacerbate the isolation and distrust often associated with mental illness.

A targeted and coordinated system of screening, referral, assessment, and diagnosis for co-occurring mental health and substance abuse disorders should be integrated into the mental health services in all jails and prisons. This approach should include active collaboration between security staff and treatment staff to share information regarding signs and symptoms of co-occurring disorders at different transition points (e.g., arrest, jail, booking, prison reception) and throughout the system. Detection of one type of disorder (i.e., substance abuse or mental illness) should immediately "trigger" investigation of the other type of disorder.

The importance of careful assessment is highlighted by the fact that one type of disorder may mimic the other, interfere with detection of the other, or overshadow the other type, and one type may actually affect the presentation of the other type of disorder.

Persons with co-occurring mental illness and substance abuse disorders who come into contact with the criminal justice system are a particularly service-intensive group. The following strategies are recommended as the most effective in treating co-occurring disorders. These strategies must be adapted for application in different settings.

- Services must be focused on the integration of treatment programming by addressing the person's mental health and substance abuse disorders simultaneously.
- Each type of disorder must be treated as primary, with a focus on understanding how they interact with each other.
- Psychosocial problems and skill deficiencies must be addressed with individualized programming, created through comprehensive assessment and consultation with the treatment participant, treatment provider, and family members.
- Medication should be prescribed with caution. Alcohol or drug use complicates or interferes with the use of prescribed medication. When circumstances warrant, an inmate not previously prescribed psychotropic medication generally should be detoxified for a reasonable period of time before psychotropic medications are prescribed unless psychotic or suicidal symptoms are present.
- Interventions must be designed for the particular setting (i.e., prisons, jails, or community corrections). Each setting requires differing intensity, length, and types of services.
- Treatment services must be extended into the community. The presence of co-occurring disorders requires special attention to discharge planning. Discharge planning is required and must address housing and job needs, family reconnection, and continued treatment.
- Treatment should be integrated with self-help groups and support networks. Support networks may be invaluable tools in assisting treatment participants in maintaining their commitment to daily alcohol and drug abstinence.

IV. HIV/AIDS

HIV and AIDS, which present extremely complex problems in the community, present even more complicated challenges in correctional settings. Among these challenges are the recognition of need for mental health services and the provision of these services. Confidentiality is complicated by the fact the there are enormous risks of social stigma and issues of personal safety that relate to the infected inmate and other inmates, as well as staff.

The usual cultural differences between the inmates and the security and health care staff may be exacerbated in cases of inmates with HIV/

AIDS because of misconceptions and fears about the illness and subculture. Education of both staff and inmates is especially important in regard to HIV/AIDS. Additionally, one public health aim of such education is to reduce the transmission risks. All inmates should have access to special educational resources dealing with prevention of transmission and consequences of continued drug use.

Housing requirements in some jurisdictions may create barriers to access to mental health treatment. Housing isolation may exacerbate the inmate's feelings of abandonment and lead to a worsening of symptoms of mental illness.

The most common psychiatric manifestations of HIV/AIDS include early signs of dementia, paranoia, and other psychotic and affective symptoms. For these reasons, it might be appropriate for a system to initiate a surveillance, outreach program, or periodic rescreening in an effort at early detection and to foster early utilization of mental health services.

The Task Force recognizes that other chronic infectious diseases, such as the group of hepatitis diseases and tuberculosis, present some of the same challenges for the delivery of psychiatric services. Therefore, many of the principles stated above may also apply to inmates with those illnesses. Further, those illnesses may be comorbid with HIV/AIDS as well as occurring alone.

V. Women

Though the number of incarcerated women in jails and prisons is small compared with the number of incarcerated men, the percentage of women compared with men incarcerated is rising, and access to psychiatric and other services is equally important. Historically, psychiatric and other treatment programs for women have been based on treatment models designed for men.

Studies show that a greater percentage of women than men entering a jail or prison setting have a serious mental illness. The rates of bipolar disorder and schizophrenia are similar for incarcerated men and women, but a larger percentage of women are diagnosed with major depression and anxiety disorders, especially posttraumatic stress disorder (PTSD).

In order to accurately diagnose and treat women with PTSD, clinicians must be trained to assess the psychological consequences of childhood and adult sexual and physical abuse. A large percentage of women (up to 70%) entering correctional settings report a history of abuse either as a child or as an adult. In addition, a higher percentage of women than men enter these settings with a history of substance abuse. Further, most women in correctional settings have at least one child for whom they have been the primary caregiver and whom they are likely to worry about during the time they are incarcerated. These issues are especially important in attending to the health care of women who are pregnant or who have given birth recently. So, for example, to minimize the risks associated with postpartum depression and psychosis, facilities should establish a policy that a comprehensive mental health evaluation be conducted whenever a woman has given birth recently.

Because of the higher prevalence of mental illness among women and their generally higher degree of willingness to participate in services, it is generally agreed that the per capita mental health staffing for female inmates needs to be significantly higher than that for men.

Clinical and corrections staff should receive training in gender-specific issues when working with female inmates. These issues must be addressed and understood in order to recognize different symptom presentation, especially among women with abuse histories. Staff and inmates also must be trained as to what constitutes sexual harassment and abuse of inmates. It is extremely important that at some point in the screening process, inmates be asked questions related to abuse histories.

The use of seclusion and restraints with women raises special concerns, because history of abuse may have involved circumstances that traumatically resonate with these interventions. As a result, these methods of control may inadvertently retraumatize inmates who have had similar experiences in the past. Some hospitals and community mental health systems have developed protocols for seclusion and restraint that involve the treatment team and the patient working together, early in the treatment process, to develop interventions that will help an agitated patient to calm down. Much of the behavior that may seem to require restraints may be de-escalated by "talking the person down" and understanding what is really going on. The behavior may be the result of dissociative phenomena or flashbacks of abuse rather than psychotic symptoms or poorly controlled impulsivity. Training is the key to understanding the behavior.

The Task Force recognizes that a substantial number of male inmates have also suffered childhood sexual abuse. Therefore, many of the aforementioned principles may also apply to them.

VI. Youth in Adult Correctional Facilities

For the purposes of these guidelines, *youth* is defined as an inmate under the age of 18. This special section is necessitated by the recent trend toward trying juveniles in adult court, which has led to an increase in the detention and incarceration of younger offenders in adult jails and prisons.

The presence of these young prisoners, who may be physically and/or emotionally less mature than their adult counterparts, has led to a plethora of challenges for correctional systems. Further, because of the selection process, in which only those juveniles charged with the most serious crimes or with the most extensive and violent criminal histories are transferred to an adult court, as a group, they are likely to be especially violent. The presence of these young prisoners in adult settings causes a number of important and challenging problems for correctional administrators. These problems include the high likelihood that they have been physically and/or sexually victimized and the real or imagined possibility of revictimization either by adults or by fellow minors. Because of their frequent immaturity and impulsivity, they also present a high risk of perpetrating violent or disruptive acts within the jail or prison environment. Also, some observers have reported high levels of neurological impairment and hyperactivity among young prisoners. These children and adolescents often face tremendous anxiety based on the uncertainties of their cases, as well as terrifying myths or fantasies about the prison experience. For convicted felons, because their sentences represent a relatively higher percentage of their life (e.g., a 16-year sentence to a 16-year-old boy is literally "life" in prison), they may perceive themselves as having "little to lose," increasing their level of dangerousness within the facility.

Some correctional systems have attempted to increase the safety of minors by requiring so-called sight and sound separation from adult prisoners. However, this response, while sensible on its face, creates barriers to programming; limits contact exclusively to other children who are equally immature, impulsive, and violent; and precludes any contact with more mature adults who might be able to model more adaptive prison behaviors. In contrast, with unsupervised access to older inmates, there is a risk that these children will be exploited or their identification with a criminal lifestyle strengthened.

Obviously, many of these challenges have tremendous implications for jail and prison mental health services. In addition to the disorders more commonly found among youth, such as attention-deficit/hyperactivity disorder (ADHD) and conduct disorders, all teenagers commonly engage in testing behaviors that are often given up by adulthood.

Because children may have limited legal ability to consent to treatment, and because many of them have "burned bridges" with their families of origin by the time they reach adult corrections, special attention must be paid to gaining legally adequate informed consent, often through the use of treatment guardians. Similarly, clinicians may have conflicting duties to inform parents about aspects of the child's care and, concomitantly, to maintain the child's confidentiality.

Because of their involvement in the juvenile and adult justice systems, these children may not have had the chance to experience the normal developmental and maturational steps. For example, if incarcerated for much of their adolescence, they may have been housed in places that do not allow any contact with opposite-gender peers.

Many of these young prisoners will have experienced severe abuse and neglect, leading to trauma-related anxiety and depressive disorders, especially PTSD, that require mental health intervention.

With or without family involvement, these young prisoners are likely to have intense psychological and social work needs relating to their families of origin. These needs may include confronting intense anger over past abuse and negotiating better relationships in the future, especially when release to family is in the near future.

The formulary, too, will have to reflect the needs of these younger patients. Pharmacies will need to reconsider the need to carry drugs that are often off-limits in adult correctional settings, such as stimulants and other medications used in mental health settings for children and youth.

As noted earlier, the likely high prevalence of neuropathology and learning disorders among this population will require access to neurological and neuropsychological evaluations and treatments, as well as special education services. Related to this, the higher impulsivity and decreased inhibition that often characterize youth predictably will cause these young prisoners to have more frequent and intense emotional crises, often including suicidal gestures or attempts, compared with adults.

A special challenge often arises when release appears imminent. Because they may never have been able to "make it on the street," or because of intense familial conflict, many young prisoners become extremely anxious, and even self-destructive, as their release date nears. Some will commit obvious and easily detectable infractions in order to forestall their own release. Mental health clinicians may be crucial in easing this transition through psychotherapy and referral to support services in the community.

Screening is no less important for children than for adults. A system should anticipate a large number of positive screens. In fact, a system may choose to presume that the factors listed herein create a presumption that each child will require some mental health assistance, and automatically treat each minor as if he or she screened positive for mental health problems. The resulting evaluation should include special attention to factors such as intelligence, history of neuropathology, special educational needs, and histories of emotional disturbances, which often may have gone undetected, thereby increasing the chances that the youth will end up in adult corrections.

Ideally, adult correctional facilities housing children should have access to mental health professionals with special education and experience in working with adolescents. At the very least, staff who work with these youths should receive specialized training in order to be able to identify emerging emotional problems and to refer the youth for treatment. They also will need special orientation to community services, if any, that will be available to the youth upon release.

It is important for correctional mental health clinicians to understand that this situation, however tragic, also presents some opportunities. For example, what may be virtually untreatable in an adult may be treatable in a teenager. Many of these children, because of learning disabilities, school truancy, expulsion, and so forth, also have severe educational deficits, that can be remedied in this literally captive population. Further, legal mandates for educational programming for children actually may increase the resources available for this population.

VII. Geriatrics and Related Issues

Effective provision of access to mental health services for older inmates in jails or prisons requires recognition of a variety of special challenges facing both inmates and mental health professionals. The National Institute of Corrections suggests that it may be useful to consider an inmate who is over the age of 50 as statistically more likely to have more common problems of "aging" even though the standard in the community is usually 65. This relatively "young" definition for the geriatric inmate population arguably may be supported by the relatively high "biological age" of an inmate because of substance abuse, including smoking, poor nutrition, lack of prior care, and generally a lower socioeconomic life in the community. The number of inmates over age 50 is increasing rapidly.

Older inmates have special medical needs that sometimes may be accompanied by psychiatric symptoms or sequelae and may complicate psychiatric intervention in terms of medication, relevance of counseling, structure of time (programming) of the inmate, and housing. The problems are more likely to be chronic, permanent, and progressive and may be related to the possibility of dying in custody. Further, treatment for these conditions may be expensive.

Special psychosocial concerns that face older inmates in jail or prison include

- Estrangement from or lack of connection to other inmates in the general population, given the relatively small (though increasing) percentage of older inmates
- Physical vulnerability to more serious consequences of assault
- More difficulty adjusting to a new environment and greater length of time needed to do so
- Higher rate of completed suicide
- Greater possibility of dying during incarceration
- Higher incidence of loss of external supports (e.g., spouse, parents, friends)

Isolation may be expressed in a variety of ways and, when extreme, may exacerbate or create mental illness or psychiatric crisis. Special issues related to isolation are acceptance after release from incarceration; provision of food, shelter, and clothing after release; assault and potentially greater sequelae of injury; and isolation from older "free" relatives and friends who themselves may be unable to travel to visit and so forth. For some of these issues, mental health intervention, including group or peer counseling, may be beneficial.

A. Terminal Illness

A *terminal illness* is defined as when death may be anticipated within a year. "Dying with dignity" is more difficult to achieve in custody. Caring for inmates with terminal illnesses may involve use of a "hospice," which may be inside the prison (less likely needed in jail) or a contract facility outside of the prison, or consideration of compassionate release. Training and written policies should be developed to address the in-custody dying inmate–patient, with consideration of the following possible plans:

1. Hospice Inside a Prison

Larger correctional systems may find it useful to house individuals together who have a likelihood of dying while in custody from an identifiable illness. A hospice inmate–patient may change in his or her ability to function physically and mentally. The hospice inmate–patient may become less oriented and behave more inappropriately as the disease and deterioration progress. Use of inmate volunteers (peer trainers) who are oriented in basic health issues, universal precautions, and mobility management may reduce the dying inmate–patient's (or his or her family's) perception that "the prison isn't doing enough."

Group therapy, realistic planning, and suicide prevention are specific interventions that the psychiatrist should either provide directly or ensure provision of by other mental health professionals.

2. Compassionate Release

Compassionate release may have a number of advantages, including cost savings for the prison health care system itself, which may be substantial. Perception of problems with public safety may decrease the viability of this option.

VIII. Mental Retardation/Developmental Disability

Offenders with co-occurring mental illness and mental retardation/developmental disability have been included as a population for which the guidelines require specialized application, because of the uniqueness of the difficulties encountered throughout the criminal justice system and treatment implications.

Mental retardation is defined as significantly subaverage intellectual functioning and impairments in adaptive functioning with onset prior to age 18. It is estimated that 40%–70% of individuals with mental retardation have diagnosable psychiatric disorders. Estimates vary widely because of the inherent difficulty in assessing behavioral manifestations of symptoms in persons with deficits in receptive and expressive language skills. Self-injurious behavior may be viewed as a manifestation of a depressive disorder, a manifestation of a diminished ability to tolerate stress, a symptom of anxiety, a problem of impulsivity, or a learned behavior leading to being the center of increased attention from others. Deficits in communication skills contribute to the difficulty in assessing the patient for psychiatrists, who depend primarily on interview and spoken language for making the correct assessment of the problem and recommending the appropriate intervention. Often, medications are prescribed to target behavioral manifestations or symptoms rather than a diagnosed underlying psychiatric disorder.

Inmates with this combination of difficulties are unfortunately the most likely to be preyed upon and ridiculed by other inmates. Their inability to process information rapidly or to comprehend instructions, their low frustration tolerance, and their impulsivity may have severe disciplinary consequences. Security and treatment staff alike must have additional training and education on mental retardation/developmental disability and clear communication in order to minimize the likelihood that behaviors will be misperceived as intentional rule infractions or attributed solely to mental retardation while a serious mental illness goes untreated. In addition, administrative, treatment, and security staff must be cognizant that the Americans With Disabilities Act is applicable to this population and make "reasonable accommodation" to the needs of these inmates.

Screening must include mechanisms to assess intellectual and adaptive functioning, as well as questions designed to elicit a history of participation in special education programs in school, and/or a history of head injury and/or seizure disorder.

The evaluation component must include the capacity to further specifically evaluate the nature and severity of limitations, either directly by facility staff or through consultation with outside providers. This may include administering individual IQ tests, assessing daily living skills, and developing a mechanism through which educational records and/or outside mental retardation/developmental disability agency service records may be secured.

Each offender's needs must be assessed individually. An offender with mental retardation may be capable of or even prefer being housed in the general population with minimal support in view of the limited choices available to inmates and the routine predictability of inmate schedules. Others, however, require additional support, protection, or scrutiny by mental health and security staff. There are a variety of ways in which provision of additional support and protection may be accomplished, including employing a specialized correctional case worker with additional training or expertise and a smaller caseload and/or placing the offender in specialized housing or programs, including continuing special education programs. Depending on the size of the population, correctional facilities or systems may choose to develop segregated housing units for inmate protection. In this instance, one must take care to ensure that offenders with mental retardation/developmental disability and mental illness are not precluded from receiving or participating in services or programs available to all other inmates.

Conclusion

We would like to take note of the fact that the authors of the 1989 guidelines set out certain precepts, which we, in this new edition of the guidelines, endorse:

> First, we take a pragmatic, rather than an "ivory tower," approach to mental health services in these settings, recognizing the constraints on the allocation of scarce resources. Second, throughout these principles we focus heavily on the phrase adequate mental health services. We use the term *adequate* rather than *minimal* to more accurately reflect the necessary level of acceptable services and to provide more leverage to obtain resources. Third, we recognize that a major obstacle to the effective delivery of mental health services is the difficult environment in which these services often must be delivered. Badly deteriorated physical plants and terrible overcrowding with highly vulnerable individuals are aspects of many jails and prisons. Moreover, even with newer physical plants and the most advanced technologies, insufficient attention to basic human needs will seriously compromise the delivery of mental health services. Unless specific attention is paid to these environments, they may negate or overwhelm therapeutic interventions and indeed all programming.
>
> Psychiatrists must define their professional responsibilities to include advocacy for improving mental health services. . . .
>
> Finally, the psychiatrist practicing in these settings is *always* bound by the standards of professional ethics as set out in the APA's Annotations Especially Applicable to Psychiatry to the AMA's Principles of Medical Ethics. These are the most fundamental statements of the moral and ethical foundations of professional psychiatric practice. (pp. 4–5)

It is in the same spirit of pragmatism informed by professional responsibility that we present this new edition of guidelines for psychiatric services in jails and prisons to our colleagues and the community.

APPENDIX

Selected Activities of the American Psychiatric Association

The publication of the second edition of these guidelines for psychiatric services in jails and prisons continues the active interest of the American Psychiatric Association (APA) in the movement to improve psychiatric services in jails and prisons.

In 1974 the APA published the following position statement:

Position Statement on Medical and Psychiatric Care in Correctional Institutions

The American Psychiatric Association recognizes that so-called correctional institutions are established by various levels of government. Their ability to provide a full range of medical (including psychiatric) services varies according to a multitude of factors: e.g., public opinion, funding, and administrative structure in relation to the goals set for a particular institution, such as punishment, containment, deterrence, rehabilitation and/or treatment.

An essential part of a minimum medical care delivery system consists of the early detection, diagnosis, treatment, and prevention of psychiatric illness. Many "correctional" facilities are not so structured as to supply this care delivery system even minimally.

It is never part of the penalty imposed to deprive a prisoner of adequate medical (including psychiatric) care. Further, it is never proper to use medical (including psychiatric) care for punitive and coercive purposes or as an instrument of social repression. The fact of incarceration imposes upon public authority the special duty to provide adequate medical services, including psychiatric services. Availability of such services is and should be a right of each incarcerated individual.

In June 1982, the Board of Trustees established the Task Force on Psychiatric Services in Correctional Facilities within the Council on Psychiatric Services. The publication, in 1989, of the first edition of these guidelines was accompanied by the following position statement:

Position Statement on Psychiatric Services in Jails and Prisons[1]

The American Psychiatric Association accords a high priority to the care and treatment of patients from groups that are underserved, especially groups that lack strong political constituencies. Such groups include the chronically mentally ill and the mentally ill homeless. Also included, but less visible, are the mentally ill in jails and prisons.

The mentally ill are especially vulnerable to the difficult conditions that typically prevail in our jails and prisons. Psychiatrists practicing in such facilities attempt to provide adequate services under the most difficult working circumstances, with inadequate professional recognition and remuneration, and, perhaps most burdensome of all, in the midst of frequently deplorable conditions.

In the 1974 "Position Statement on Medical and Psychiatric Care in Correctional Institutions," APA called for a "full range of . . . psychiatric services" in jails and prisons. Noting that "an essential part of a minimal medical care delivery system consists of the early detection, diagnosis, treatment, and prevention of psychiatric illness," the APA position statement went on to forcefully state that "the fact of incarceration imposes upon public authority the special duty to provide adequate medical services, including psychiatric services. Availability of such services is and should be a right of the incarcerated individual."

However, a decade later, in 1983, APA was obliged to observe that "providing mental health treatment for persons in jails and prisons has, over the years, proved a refractory problem, . . . [with reasons cited]" In part, this situation persists because of the altered social context of the operations of correctional facilities, which has resulted in tightened admission criteria for psychiatric hospitalization, fewer beds, limits on length of stay, reduced availability and use of civil commitments, and changing sentencing practices that have increased the number of inmates needing mental health services. Legislative demands for fiscal austerity and associated public policies, such as deinstitutionalization, have led to a complex set of circumstances that have been associated with an increase in the number of mentally ill persons who are at risk of incarceration in local jails because of minor charges used to address their disturbed behavior. This situation has resulted in a substantial increase in the population of inmates requiring mental health care.

Severe overcrowding is an additional factor often contributing to the inadequacy of psychiatric services in jails and prisons. Conditions are often so bad in today's jails and prisons that both state and federal courts have mandated sweeping changes in their operations. The Supreme Court has ruled that it is the obligation of correctional officials

---

[1]American Psychiatric Association, Task Force on Psychiatric Services in Correctional Facilities: "Position Statement on Psychiatric Services in Jails and Prisons." *American Journal of Psychiatry* 146:1244, 1989.

to ensure that the civil rights of inmates and detainees with mental illness are protected. This obligation includes the right to adequate mental health care. Providing adequate mental health care in this context rests on the following principles:

1. The fundamental goal of a mental health service should be to provide the same level of care to patients in the criminal justice process that is available in the community.
2. The effective delivery of mental health services in correctional settings requires that there be a recognition that security and treatment are mutually dependent. There is no inherent conflict between security and treatment.
3. A therapeutic environment can be created in a jail or a prison setting if there is clinical leadership and adequate resource with authority to create such an environment.
4. Timely and effective access to mental health treatment is a hallmark of adequate mental health care. Necessary staffing levels should be determined by what is essential to ensure that access.
5. Psychiatrists should take a leadership role administratively as well as clinically. Further, it is imperative that psychiatrists define their professional responsibilities to include advocacy for improving mental health services in jails and prisons.
6. Psychiatrists should actively oppose discrimination based on religion, race, ethnic background, or sexual preference, not only for mental health services but for all activities in the judicial-legal process.

Elaborations and explications of these principles can be found in the report of the Task Force on Psychiatric Services in Jails and Prisons, June 1988, which will be available from the APA Office of Psychiatric Services in the near future.

Finally, APA calls on its members to participate in the care and treatment of the mentally ill in jails and prisons, for without an increased commitment and involvement of its membership in providing services to the mentally ill in jails and prisons, position statements such as this will be meaningless. The breadth and depth of these problems demand much more.

This new position statement was accompanied by the following editorial in the same issue of *The American Journal of Psychiatry*[2]:

---

[2] Weinstein HC: "Psychiatric Services in Jails and Prisons: Who Cares?" (editorial). *American Journal of Psychiatry* 146:1094–1095, 1989.

Psychiatric Services in Jails and Prisons: Who Cares?

On any day, our nation's jails and prisons hold an estimated 1.2 million men and women. Many studies have consistently demonstrated that about 20% of these inmates are seriously mentally ill and in need of psychiatric care. Up to 5% are actively psychotic. What constitutes psychiatric care for these people? Who will care for these people? Who cares?

In the Official Actions section of this issue of the journal is a position statement developed by the APA Task Force on Psychiatric Services in Jails and Prisons and approved by the Assembly of District Branches and the Board of Trustees. It reaffirms that "the American Psychiatric Association accords a high priority to the care and treatment of patients from groups that are underserved, especially groups that lack strong political constituencies. Such groups include the chronically mentally ill and the mentally ill homeless. Also included, but less visible, are the mentally ill in jails and prisons."

This position statement traces APA's concern for the mentally ill in jails and prisons over the past two decades, rejecting an "out of sight, out of mind" mentality and the unstated dynamic that medical and psychiatric neglect should be a part of the criminal justice process of retribution and punishment.

And yet, in what many regard as difficult days for psychiatry, these issues are far from the active concerns of the average psychiatric practitioner. This is understandable, but what about the responsibility of the profession? What about our ideals of public service?

On the other hand, in these often problematic settings, where almost all of psychiatry's problems are raised to a higher power, is the attempt to bring quality psychiatric care to these patients a cruel joke? Where serious political and economic problems are the rule (such as harsh questions of the allocation of very scarce resources and grossly inadequate remuneration), is this the time or the place for "pie in the sky"?

Then, of course, there are the subtle (and sometimes not so subtle) ethical conflicts: informed consent in these settings, confidentiality (are you kidding?), and divided loyalties, not to mention the unexamined countertransference. Is it any wonder that some may say, "Who needs it?"

Well, we need it. In a time of profound internal professional questioning and external competition, what better way to adopt an active leadership stance and develop and maintain the highest standards of practice? What better test of our goal of bringing quality care to the needy? What better challenge to our ideals, our resolve? What better way to play a major part in reforming this neglected aspect of our health and mental health care delivery system?

The position statement sets out a number of principles:

1. The fundamental goal of a mental health service should be to provide the same level of care to patients in the criminal justice process that is available in the community.
2. The effective delivery of mental health services in correctional settings requires that there be a balance between security and treatment needs. There is no inherent conflict between security and treatment.
3. A therapeutic environment can be created in a jail or a prison setting if there is clinical leadership, with authority to create such an environment.
4. Timely and effective access to mental health treatment is a hallmark of adequate mental health care. Necessary staffing levels should be determined by what is essential to ensure that access.
5. Psychiatrists should take a leadership role administratively as well as clinically. Further, it is imperative that psychiatrists define their professional responsibilities to include advocacy for improving mental health service in jails and prisons.

The specific objectives that are required to meet these goals are set out in the report of the task force, which also has been recently approved by the Board of Trustees. This document is made up of two parts. The first part, "Principles Governing the Delivery of Psychiatric Services in Jails and Prisons," deals with such issues as the quality of care, confidentiality, informed consent, research, and treatment as well as administration and administrative issues, education and training, and interprofessional relationships. It calls for more training in correctional psychiatry at the residency level and increased efforts by academic departments to reach out to correctional facilities in order to establish affiliations for the provision of services, education, and research.

The second part of the task force report, "Guidelines for Psychiatric Services in Jails and Prisons," provides specific standards for the delivery of essential psychiatric services in the three major types of facilities: lockups, jails, and prisons. For each type of facility, services are grouped under four categories: screening and evaluation, crisis intervention, treatment, and discharge/transfer planning. The latter section responds to the fact that efforts to develop community resources to support the reintegration of a mentally ill population back into society are even more pervasively problematical in correctional psychiatry than they are in public psychiatry in general.

Finally, it is important to note that these principles and guidelines supplement the standards set out by the National Commission on Correctional Health Care. This commission, which grew out of an American Medical Association–sponsored consortium of national health care organizations, including APA, whose members provide health care services in jails and prisons, has developed an excellent set of standards and a highly regarded accreditation process. That the APA guidelines are thus based on and complementary to American Medical Association–derived standards of practice is consistent with the remedicalization of psychiatry.

APA's "Position Statement on Psychiatric Services in Jails and Prisons" is, most of all, a call to action: a call for the participation of the members of APA in this important public service. By adopting this position statement and the principles and guidelines for psychiatric services in jails and prisons, APA emphatically asserts that it cares and that psychiatrists should and will in the future be a substantial presence in these settings.

Having completed the principal aspects of its charge, the Task Force recommended to the APA that a regular committee of the APA be formed to continue this work.

In 1990 the Committee on Psychiatric Services in Jails and Prisons was created. This committee provided a locus of activity for the APA in this area. The committee provided courses and programs and established contacts with other interested individuals and groups.

The reorganization of the APA Council on Psychiatric Services led to changing the committee from a free-standing entity to a voting component of the Consortium on Special Delivery Settings of the Council.

In turn, members of the APA who felt the need for a special group representing correctional psychiatry formed the Caucus of Psychiatrists Practicing in Criminal Justice Settings. This effort has received the strong support of the APA Council on Psychiatric Services and the Board of Trustees. At the time of the writing of these guidelines, the Board of Trustees of the APA had allocated a grant for the development and recruitment efforts of the Caucus of Psychiatrists Practicing in Criminal Justice Settings.

Suggested Readings

It is suggested that the following publications be consulted. These readings each include extensive references and bibliographies.

Anno J: *Prison Health Care: Guidelines for the Management of an Adequate Delivery System.* Chicago, IL, National Commission on Correctional Health Care, 1991

Cohen F: *The Mentally Disordered Inmate and the Law.* Kingston, NJ, Civic Research Institute, 1998

Metzner JL: "An Introduction to Correctional Psychiatry, Part I." *Journal of the American Academy of Psychiatry and Law* 25:375–381, 1997

Metzner JL: "An Introduction to Correctional Psychiatry, Part II." *Journal of the American Academy of Psychiatry and Law* 25:571–579, 1997

Metzner JL: "An Introduction to Correctional Psychiatry, Part III." *Journal of the American Academy of Psychiatry and Law* 26:107–115, 1998

National Commission on Correctional Health Care: *Standards for Health Services in Jails.* Chicago, IL, National Commission on Correctional Health Care, 1996

National Commission on Correctional Health Care: *Standards for Health Services in Prisons.* Chicago, IL, National Commission on Correctional Health Care, 1997

Wettstein R (ed): *Treatment of Offenders with Mental Disorders.* New York, Guilford, 1998

Index